THE
GREAT
CARDIO
MYTH

WHY CARDIO EXERCISE WON'T GET YOU SLIM, STRONG, OR HEALTHY—**AND THE NEW HIGH-INTENSITY STRENGTH TRAINING PROGRAM THAT WILL**

Craig Ballantyne, CTT, M.Sc., creator of Turbulence Training

with Chelsea Ratcliff

FAIR WINDS

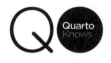

Quarto is the authority on a wide range of topics.

Quarto educates, entertains and enriches the lives of our readers—enthusiasts and lovers of hands-on living.

www.QuartoKnows.com

First published in the United States of America in 2017 by
Fair Winds Press, an imprint of
Quarto Publishing Group USA Inc.
100 Cummings Center
Suite 406-L
Beverly, Massachusetts 01915-6101
Telephone: (978) 282-9590
Fax: (978) 283-2742
QuartoKnows.com
Visit our blogs at QuartoKnows.com

21 20 19 18 17   1 2 3 4 5

ISBN: 978-1-59233-739-2

Library of Congress Cataloging-in-Publication Data is available.

Design and Page Layout: Megan Jones Design
Photography: Clarkson Creative, Trevor Brown

Printed in China

The information in this book is for educational purposes only. It is not intended to replace the advice of a physician or medical practitioner. Please see your health-care provider before beginning any new health program.

CONTENTS

FOREWORD

IF YOU'VE EVER had the feeling you were wasting your time . . . if you ever felt like "going to the gym" was just a big joke on you . . . if you ever looked in the mirror and thought with despair, *What the heck was the point of the forty hours I spent on the treadmill over the last three months?* Prepare to be enlightened about cardio exercise.

You'll see how giving up cardio—and taking a little-known but faster path—can not only help you achieve your fat loss goals but also improve your health in a number of ways.

Despite weight loss being the number one goal of most people who join a gym, creating exercise programs to help people lose belly fat is actually a new concept. To be honest, it simply wasn't needed in the past. People were more active and, overall, moved more than they do today.

Today, in an almost completely automated time-crunched society, we, as exercise professionals, have had to create exercise programs specifically to induce fat loss. Designing exercise specifically for fat loss has led to a number of trial-and-error theories, methods, and concepts that, in the end, have been unsuccessful.

As a fitness industry we have failed miserably.

We originally designed fat loss programs by copying what endurance athletes were doing and hoping that, somehow, the training program of a marathon runner would work for fat loss—even when we cut it down to twenty minutes, three times per week. But fat loss was never the goal of endurance athletes—it was a side effect. Standing at the finish line of any marathon you'll see bodies of all shapes and sizes able to cross, proving that running a marathon doesn't always equal fat loss.

Fitness experts also turned to bodybuilding for ideas about fat loss. This was in the 1980s when physique transformation contests became so popular. Average people underwent strenuous bodybuilding regimens to produce startling changes in their appearance—à la Arnold Schwarzenegger. But to take the programs of full-time bodybuilders and use them to model fat loss programs for the general population was nonsensical, and, perhaps, not the healthiest.

But we tried.

And the nutritional supplement companies jumped right on board to try to convince us that taking Brand X powders, pills, and shakes would provide the same benefits as the drugs that bodybuilders were using.

We failed again. Rates of obesity remained high and overall fitness levels were not improving. Cardiovascular diseases were not declining at nearly the rate it seemed they should.

But we were getting closer. Fat loss was indeed a goal for bodybuilders, but the low levels of body fat percentage a contest bodybuilder achieved was a result of increased muscle mass and, therefore, metabolism (and training programs several hours in length per day)—not from lots of steady-state cardio.

With the simplicity of an aerobic workout, and the media hype surrounding it, many people, instead, turned to cardio to try to improve their fitness and lose weight.

Then we discovered the truth: Aerobic work really doesn't do much for fat loss. Scientific study after scientific study shows little to no fat loss with aerobic programs.

Steady-state aerobic exercise for fat loss might be the biggest lie ever told in the fitness industry. Cardio work can improve cardiovascular fitness, and fit athletes tend to be lean. But even though there was a correlation between cardiovascular fitness and leanness, there was never cause and effect. Adding cardio exercise—particularly aerobic work—doesn't translate to any meaningful fat loss results.

A 1998 study showed that the addition of forty-five minutes of aerobic exercise at 78 percent max heart rate five days a week for twelve weeks had *no effect* over dieting alone.[1]

A 2007 study looked at a six-month period of time with two groups: diet only versus diet plus aerobic exercise (this time for fifty minutes, five days per week).[2] This study concluded there is no additional effect of aerobic exercise on body composition.

And another 2007 study looked at an even longer duration—twelve months.[3] In addition, there was a longer workout period—sixty minutes instead of forty-five or fifty—and an extra day per week (six days as opposed to five).

This time, though, the program worked—sort of.

The average fat loss for the year was around a measly three and a half pounds (1.6 kg).

As you'll see in these and other studies covered in this book, aerobics for fat loss is not an effective use of time.

This is where Craig Ballantyne comes in. Craig has the scientific background to actually dig deep into the research and look at what worked and what didn't. Craig also walks the walk (or in his case, sprints the sprint) and is a real-world practitioner, training real people and getting them to see real results that match what scientists have achieved in the exercise labs. Over the last fifteen-plus years, Craig has refined and developed a fat loss methodology featured in dozens of magazines all over the world.

He's about to show you a more modern and feasible exercise path to disease prevention, functional fitness, and improved well-being—the health benefits we were once told we could only get through hours of cardio.

Even though we are fitness experts and gym owners and have written six books on exercise, we still learn something from Craig every time we speak with him. He's not only a walking, talking billboard for his methods, he's also a truth-telling inspiration to millions . . . and you're about to get his latest secrets, along with a guided tour of the research that reveals why they work.

—Alwyn and Rachel Cosgrove, Results Fitness

INTRODUCTION

I HAVE AN EMBARRASSING story to tell you. In my second year of college, I fell for the "cardio myth"—hook, line, and sinker. I was already a young, strong athlete on a competitive soccer team, but I thought adding more cardio to my training would help me "get ripped" and improve my fitness; instead it turned me from a 180-pound (81.5 kg) muscular young man into a 160-pound (72.5 kg) sand-kicked-in-my-face weakling suffering from overuse injuries.

At first I was confused. Weren't all these miles logged on the road supposed to give me six-pack abs and get me in peak shape?

Fortunately, that mistake lasted just one summer. The next year at school, I rebuilt my fitness-model body with strength training. I got leaner, stronger, and more attractive.

You might even say I got smarter because this lesson inspired me to earn a graduate degree in exercise science at McMaster University in Hamilton, Ontario. I wanted to understand why and how exercise led to optimal health. Yes, *health*, because having too much body fat and too little muscle are obviously not just a matter of "looks." An overly fat, flabby physique links to myriad health risks—from heart disease to diabetes to osteoporosis and injuries.

As I started to examine the effects of exercise, I realized how complex the science behind it was and how detrimental some common assumptions about cardio might be, not just for athletes, but for the general public, as well.

In 1999, the year before I graduated, I developed my own training program based on the research coming out at the time, combined with my own experience. I called it Turbulence Training (you'll see why in chapter 4). I've spent the last two decades continuing to study exercise myths and scientifically proven breakthroughs, thus helping hundreds of thousands of men and women kick cardio to the curb for good and sculpt a slimmer, sexier body with short burst exercise sessions.

The "short burst" concept increasingly caught the attention of journalists, including my coauthor, Chelsea Ratcliff. Back in 2011, Chelsea interviewed me for a *U.S. News* story about the major ways women were wasting time at the gym. Given her additional academic work in health communication, she was the right person to help me expose how myths get started.

This book pulls the curtain back on a number of myths about cardiovascular exercise, so you won't make the same mistakes I did. Some of these myths are minor, while others are, as the science shows, quite serious and potentially injurious. All surely contribute to the current struggle of many Americans to achieve good health, not to mention maintain a healthy body weight—a challenge that persists despite a burgeoning $60 billion weight-loss market!

On a personal note, it is also my mission to stop guys my age from dropping dead in marathons. It happens almost every month, and these men are leaving widows and kids behind in the quest for worthless participation medals.

The myths we discuss have been decades in the making, even though ever-widening waistlines, and the chronic diseases that come with them, should have been our first clue that cardio, America's favorite exercise, might not be all it's cracked up to be.

For years, we've been told that to **lose weight**, we have to do endurance exercise.

We've been told that for **cardiovascular health and longevity**, long cardio sessions are the only answer.

As I discovered, and you'll see for yourself in this book, both are false. In fact, new research is showing us that, in large doses, cardio exercise might not even be safe.

The government, the media, and weight-loss professionals have all stepped in to address the American—even global—obesity crisis, and exercise is part of their prescription. But they're largely propagating the very cardio concepts—outdated and disproven—that have failed to work.

And it's not just the Average Joe and Jane who fall for this stuff. It is exercise scientists, personal trainers, doctors, health advocates, and even athletes like me. Some people literally get addicted to cardio in pursuit of health and fitness, and it leads them into black holes of exercise punctuated by injuries that render them couch-bound and depressed, sometimes creating a cycle of weight loss and weight gain.

One of the most tragic examples of this can be seen in the aftermath of the popular reality TV show *The Biggest Loser*. Each season, obese men and women lose *hundreds* of pounds, only to gain much of the weight back within a few years. Some end up heavier than before they started.

A recent study published in the journal *Obesity* tracked a group of fourteen contestants from *The Biggest Loser* for up to six years after their appearance on the TV show.[4] The study, backed by the National Institutes of Health (NIH), found that thirteen of the fourteen participants couldn't keep the weight off—and not for lack of trying. Season 8 winner Danny Cahill devoted hours a day to exercise, and even quit his job trying to hold on to his victory.[5] He started his day on the treadmill at 5 a.m., rode his bike to the gym (where he did even more cardio), and ended his day with a night run. But, as he told the *New York Times*, he battled increasingly fierce food cravings and an ever-slowing metabolism. According to the *Obesity* study, he now burns 800 fewer calories per day than expected for a man his size.

These *Biggest Loser* contestants lose astonishing amounts of weight through extreme diet and exercise. They exercise for up to seven hours a day, including lots and lots of cardio, and after the show is over, they are advised to exercise at least nine hours a week to maintain their results. Nine hours a week! But hours of cardio a day didn't prevent Danny from regaining one hundred pounds (45 kg).

Weight regain is a complex phenomenon, and I wouldn't go so far as to say it's *all* cardio's fault. But I believe cardio is a big part of it.

So, what is cardio? It is long, low- to medium-intensity, repetitive endurance activities. These activities include running, jogging, walking, cycling, elliptical machines, stationary bikes, and aerobics.

Most people don't lose weight with steady-state cardio; for those who do, the results are usually fleeting. That's because people who do a high volume of cardio often:

- Lose muscle mass, which slows your metabolism and, ultimately, makes it harder to lose fat (very likely the main culprit behind the slowed metabolisms of *The Biggest Loser* contestants); or

- Get injured (up to 70 percent of runners suffer an overuse injury each year, according to research); or

- Realize that 300 minutes of cardio is pretty much impossible for anyone with a job, family, or social life (let alone all three) and quit.

If you're like me, you have a lot you want to accomplish in life. You may want to raise a family, have a successful career, and enjoy your free time. No doubt you want to be healthy, too, but not at the expense of all your other life goals.

Having good health and fitness should not require a massive sacrifice. Nor should your pursuit of health leave you worse off than when you started. So why go down that rabbit hole?

Clearly, *The Biggest Loser* approach of high volumes of cardio and drastic dieting—which has been the standard weight loss approach in the United States for decades—is not the best answer. In fact, it appears to be exactly the wrong answer.

Today, the tide is shifting away from cardio exercise toward my beloved strength training and metabolic resistance training workouts (like you get in Turbulence Training). But still, far too many people rely on cardio machines thinking it will get them fit, toned, and skinny. Why is that, despite all the research that proves it doesn't work, it leads to injury, and, in some cases, serious health issues? Because cardio is the brain-dead easy-way-out for exercise. It's like the fast food of the fitness world. All you have to do is put one foot in front of the other and you can go for a jog. Or plop your butt on a stationary bike and slowly pedal away while reading a magazine. But that doesn't mean it's going to do anything for you. After all, it's called the easy way out, not the easy way to success.

Strength training, on the other hand, is, I admit, a little intimidating. However, it works much better, much faster, and for many more attributes of fitness. Not only can you improve your cardiovascular fitness and health with strength training, but you can also fight diabetes, boost your bone strength, and lose belly fat while adding muscle mass and strength.

Unfortunately, most people don't know where to start. Well, fear not. In addition to proving why cardio is a big waste of time, you'll also discover how to do strength training workouts with dumbbells and bodyweight exercises that give you more energy, get you back in shape, and boost your sex appeal to your partner . . . or person you'd like to have as your partner. So skip your jog, sit back, and enjoy this journey as you discover the truth about what really works in the exercise world.

Perhaps the greatest damage done by the cardio myths is that, because of them, many people are not exercising at all.

As you're about to see, there is a better way to reap the benefits of being active. Research increasingly suggests that as little as four minutes of intense exercise could replace a thirty-, sixty-, or ninety-minute cardio session. The *New York Times* even reported that a one-minute burst of intense exercise flanked by a few minutes of warm-up and cool-down was as good as forty-five minutes of aerobic exercise.[6] Short bursts of intense exercise can replace hours of cardio and deliver the same, sometimes better, health rewards. You'll learn more about the research behind this concept later.

For years, people have been slogging the miles, wearing through their running shoes, and buying pair after pair . . . even buying orthotics and braces to deal with injuries acquired along the way.

After reading this book, my guess is that some avid runners, cyclists, and other endurance athletes will decide to scale back their training. Recreational exercisers will be thrilled to discover they can get the same—actually, better—health and fitness results in much less time than a typical cardio session, without many of the risks. And yes, some cardio addicts will send me hate mail. Or would, if they had any time to write it.

Perhaps the greatest damage done by the cardio myths is that, because of them, many people are not exercising at all. Those who hate repetitive exercise, who gave up after a lack of results, or who simply don't have time for the long sessions they've been *told* are necessary are forever putting off exercise for "tomorrow." This is the catch-22 of cardio.

But now you have a choice. You can remain stuck in the cardio matrix, or you can break free and finally get results. The choice is yours. And now you have an educated guide to show you the way.

—Craig Ballantyne

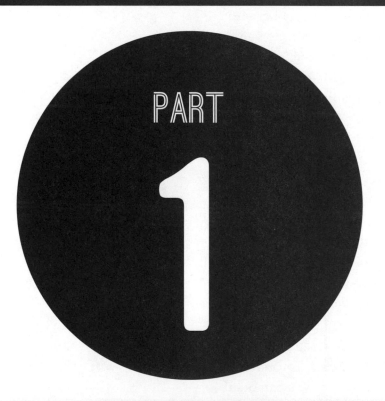

PART

1

THE
MAJOR
MYTHS

18,720 minutes
of aerobic exercise
=
4 to 6 pounds
(1.8 to 2.7 kg)
of weight loss*

*This is based on a recommendation of 312 hours—or 18,720 minutes—per year (see page 22).

RUNNING THE WRONG WAY:

HOW AMERICA WAS FOOLED BY THE CULT OF CARDIO

I N 1960, JOHN F. KENNEDY wrote an editorial for *Sports Illustrated* titled "The Soft American." He warned that physical activity was being "engineered" out of daily life at an alarming pace.[7]

It was the price for modern conveniences. The typical American was now desk-bound by day and huddled around the TV at night. As for "exercise," many people considered it the realm of athletes and military trainees. The result: some folks were getting scrawny; many more were getting fat. And the wheezing and growing waistlines appeared to be linked to worsening health.

We were headed for a public health crisis, and president-elect Kennedy sounded the alarm: Our spreading sedentariness could "undermine our capacity for thought" and even be "a menace to our security." He went so far as to say, "Such softness on the part of individual citizens can help strip and destroy the vitality of a nation."

Kennedy declared it was time for the United States to launch a nationwide effort to fix our fitness fiasco. Not long after, a young military doctor from Oklahoma would propose a solution.

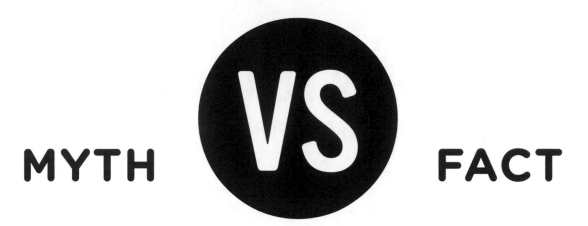

MYTH VS FACT

Myth	Fact
Early studies found that cardio keeps the heart healthy and adds years to life.	Early studies found heart health and longevity benefits from *all* types of physical activity!
Strength training is an inessential "extra" and takes a backseat to endurance exercise.	Strength training is a critical component of an exercise regimen because it preserves muscle mass, keeping metabolism up and helping prevent injury.
Plenty of research shows that cardio helps people lose fat.	A closer look at the data usually reveals minimal weight loss, and sometimes it is loss of muscle weight rather than body fat.
Sixty minutes of exercise a day is required to stave off fat gain.	With the right kinds of exercise, you can lose fat and keep it off with much shorter workouts—as little as three, twenty-minute sessions per week (or fewer!).

In the mid-1960s, a physician named Kenneth Cooper began developing a physical conditioning program for NASA and the U.S. Air Force. The training program would ensure that astronauts' and airmen's hearts and lungs were in top condition before flight. The program seemed like it could help the general population improve physical fitness, too, so he decided to let the public in on his groundbreaking invention. The invention? Aerobics.

Dr. Cooper published *Aerobics* in 1968 and the book was a hit. He was playing off the term "aerobic," which means, "requiring free oxygen," to describe physical activities that use a great deal of oxygen and can be done continuously. The benefit, he said, was improved cardiorespiratory fitness—perhaps even protection against heart disease. To stay fit, according to Cooper, one simply needed to do a certain amount of aerobic exercise every week. His top five activities were running (or jogging), cycling, swimming, cross-country skiing, and walking.

Here was physical activity for the masses. Aerobics was thought to be safe, low-impact, and easy. Now anyone, regardless of age or sex, could exercise. Families could exercise together, and they did.

The number of exercisers in the United States doubled in a decade: "According to the Gallup Poll, 24 percent of American adults exercised regularly in 1961, and 50 percent after 1968," Cooper told the *New York Times*.[8] Without a doubt, his program had helped get Americans moving.

In 1970, Dr. Cooper founded the Cooper Institute for Aerobics Research in Texas. A year later, he opened the Cooper Aerobics Center, a mansion-turned-fitness-center that would later include a hotel and spa. Businessmen and dignitaries flocked here to get in shape. In 1988, future president George W. Bush even did.[9]

When Cooper's aerobics program was credited with helping the 1970 Brazilian soccer team win the World Cup, his popularity spread around the globe, and his aerobics books were translated into forty-one languages.[10] The cardio-as-preventive-medicine concept was now "common knowledge."

MORE REASONS TO LACE UP OUR NIKES

The early data from Dr. Cooper and his colleagues seemed promising. Aerobics apparently had the potential to add years to our lives—not to mention make us feel more alive. A daily run could offer revitalizing stress relief and relaxation, Dr. Cooper explained. And while promises of vitality (and even virility) were anecdotal, his team did present data to back up the longevity benefits.

Pilot studies had identified a possible link between physical fitness and lower coronary risk factors[11], and, in 1989, the Cooper Institute finally had enough empirical data to make a full-fledged case for it. The Institute's pioneering longitudinal study of over 13,000 participants was published by the *Journal of the*

American Medical Association (*JAMA*), and results showed a clear relationship between physical fitness and reduced mortality.[12] The fitter participants seemed less susceptible not only to heart disease but also to cancer, the study found. The link between fitness and longer life was independent of other risk factors, including smoking and cholesterol level; those suspected of having a preexisting condition were excluded from the participant pool. Get active, live longer. It was as simple as that.

The popularity of aerobic activities soared in the 1970s and 1980s. Dr. Cooper was known as "the man who got America running" and even started a worldwide jogging craze.[13] Jim Fixx, Dr. George Sheehan, and Brian Maxwell joined the list of running evangelists whose books touted benefits from stress relief to better sex to the euphoric "runner's high."

By 1982, Dr. Cooper had written four books: the seminal 1968 *Aerobics* and three follow-ups. These guides were based on a points-based system for achieving the ultimate level of aerobic fitness, and together they sold twelve million copies.[14]

The media broadcasted Cooper's pro-cardio message to living rooms everywhere. He was invited to speak on *Good Morning America* and *The Today Show*, and major newspapers from the *Chicago Sun-Times* to the *Tribune* in San Diego and *Star Tribune* in Minneapolis clamored for interviews.[15] In 1987, a journalist for the *New York Times* cheered: "Over the last two decades, America has been swept by a fitness and exercise boom that

EXERCISE 101

When I talk about *cardio*, I am referring to the standard conceptualization of it: aerobic exercise done at a steady or continuous pace, also sometimes called "endurance activity." The most common examples include cycling, running, and walking.

Interval exercise typically uses a cardio activity, such as cycling, but with a varying level of intensity. With *high-intensity intermittent exercise* (HIIE), you alternate short bursts of anaerobic exercise with very low-intensity aerobic exercise. Another term for this is *high-intensity interval training*, or HIIT.

The other main type of exercise is *strength training*. This uses movements with added resistance created either with weights or your bodyweight. Some newer HIIT protocols incorporate strength exercises with interval cardio, and some are even completely resistance focused.

has taken on almost religious fervor. Joggers, swimmers, cyclists, and skiers are everywhere, spreading the word."[16]

"If this movement has a high priest," the journalist wrote, "it is Dr. Kenneth H. Cooper."[17]

Following an aerobics program would award you with vitality, heart health, and a longer life, the news reported. All you had to do was lace up your trainers and go.[18]

For those who preferred not to run, there was aerobic dance, which soon had millions of women (and Richard Simmons) donning spandex leotards, legwarmers, and contrasting tights. The recipe for results was the same:

duration
(the longer, the better)

+

intensity
(something sustainable for an hour or more)

+

frequency
(at least three times a week—ideally every day)

Adhering to these guidelines—and a steady choreography of "grapevines" and toe taps—was supposed to give you a safe, low-impact way to "get the blood circulating." With any luck, you might even come out looking like Jane Fonda, the high priestess of the VHS aerobics movement.

Following an aerobics program would award you with vitality, heart health, and longer life, the news reported. All you had to do was lace up your trainers and go.

AFTER FIVE DECADES OF CARDIO: WHERE ARE WE NOW?

Fifty years after it first pulled Americans out of their chairs, aerobics is still the go-to fitness activity. We know it as cardiovascular activity, or just "cardio," but the definition is the same: long, steady-state endurance activity.

Running is more popular than ever, though Fixx, Sheehan, Maxwell, and many champions of endurance running have passed away (some, quite tragically, while running). In 2013, nineteen million Americans participated in running events.[19] The number of marathoners and 5k-ers is at a steady incline, and that's just the hardcore folk; a whopping sixty-five million Americans consider themselves regular runners or joggers.[20]

Here is a typical gym-goer's routine: punching the clock on a treadmill or elliptical machine, or saddling up on a stationary bike, and zoning out for thirty to sixty minutes. Dance workout classes still fill up (Zumba has replaced Jazzercise) and Jane Fonda is, incredibly, still making workout videos. With near cult-level worship of cardio, you'd think we'd be in pretty good shape by now—but we aren't.

In fact, after fifty years of cardio, America is fatter and unhealthier than ever before. Far from the "vital populace" that Kennedy envisioned and aerobics promised to deliver, we've gone from "soft" to a complete health meltdown. Two-thirds of American adults today are overweight, and a full one-third are considered obese, the Centers for Disease

Control and Prevention (CDC) reports.[21] Complications from obesity and inactivity together take 365,000 lives each year, making this the second-leading behavioral cause of death in the United States. (The only thing worse is smoking.)[22]

As obesity rates continue to climb, obesity and inactivity may surpass tobacco as the number one behavioral cause of death in America.[23] Heart disease now causes one in four deaths in the United States, claiming more than 600,000 lives a year.[24] And, finally, despite their daily runs, many Americans are still stressed, depressed, and exhausted.[25]

This means either most Americans still aren't exercising, or, more likely, they're not exercising "enough" to stave off weight gain, heart disease, and psychological unease. So why hasn't cardio saved us, like it promised to do?

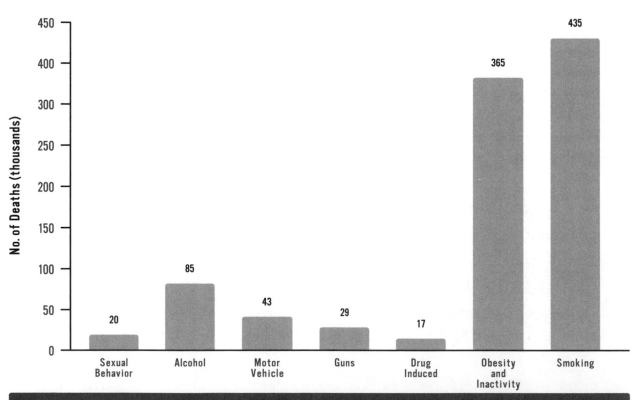

U.S. DEATHS FROM BEHAVIORAL CAUSES[22]
Figure 1.1: Number of U.S. Deaths from Behavioral Causes in 2000

HOW SIXTY-FIVE MILLION PEOPLE COULD BE WRONG

It's a tough pill to swallow. I was incredulous myself, but there was no way to hide from the evidence any longer: Cardio wasn't living up to its claims. After digging deeper, I came to the same conclusion so many other exercise scientists have: Cardiovascular activity is only one part of the exercise puzzle—and a much smaller part than we were led to believe.

In reality, long, steady-state cardio is neither essential for heart health nor effective for weight loss. It doesn't properly prepare you for functional aging, and it can make you weaker and reduce your ability to produce power. This is certainly not the first time the government, media, doctors, and celebrities have rallied behind a cause that missed the mark. Remember low-fat diets?

Since the invention of aerobics in the 1960s, the benefits of cardio have been understudied, over reported, hyped up by journalists, promoted by stakeholders, and even, in some cases, purely imagined. I don't believe the claims were made with any malicious intent. They were based on the research available at the time . . . though the study designs may have been flawed, the results cherry-picked, and research groups, such as the Cooper Institute, holding clear conflicts of interest.

Despite decades of research showing that other forms of exercise trump cardio for weight loss and other benefits, the cardio myths have continued to flourish. It's high time someone shouted, "The emperor has no clothes!" and pulled back the curtain on the numerous myths about cardiovascular activity. We can start by revealing the so-called empirical evidence, woven by scientists eager to claim their study effects were significant.

A CLOSER LOOK AT THE CARDIO RESEARCH

When Catherine signed up for my training program, she had been trying for years to lose weight. A forty-four-year-old mother and former actress living in California, she wanted her younger, pre-pregnancy figure back. But like so many, she thought she needed a rigorous cardio regimen to get it.

Catherine tried step aerobics, spinning, and running on the treadmill. She devoted hours to cardio each week, but, throughout her late thirties and early forties, the excess body fat barely budged. Though she managed through great effort to get down to 165 pounds (75 kg), on her small 5'1" (155 cm) frame, this was still considered clinically obese.

Eventually, Catherine caught on—and if you've been at it for a while now, you probably have too. The link between cardio and weight loss ain't what it's cracked up to be. Yet here people are, logging miles, counting "calories burned" on their machines, and squandering precious hours in the name of cardio. Taking a magnifying glass to the scientific literature could have saved us all the trouble.

Let's start with a 2007 study published in the journal *Obesity* that *did* find weight loss benefits from cardio.[26]

How much cardio? Sixty minutes per day.

How much weight loss? After one year, four to six pounds (1.8 to 2.7 kg).

You might want to reread that.

I had to because I couldn't believe my eyes: In twelve months of moderate to vigorous aerobic activity, six days a week, for one hour per day, previously sedentary women only lost four pounds (1.8 kg) and just 1.4 cm (½ inch) off their waists. Men in the study fared slightly better, losing roughly six and a half pounds (3 kg) and 3.3 cm (1.3 inches) off their waists.

An effect was only observed, mind you, for those who did at least 250 minutes of cardio per week. That's about 4.2 hours each week, or 218 hours per year, *minimum*. To get the full sixty minutes a day, six days a week, per the study protocol, you're looking at 312 hours per year.

What these researchers failed to acknowledge was that you can get better fat loss results from high-intensity interval exercise (HIIE) in twenty minutes a day, three times a week.[27] You can even get heart health benefits from HIIE.[28] An interval workout regimen (like those included in this book) would add up to just seventy-eight hours per year, leaving you with 234 hours leftover—enough time for a nine-day vacation.

Perhaps the strangest aspect of the *Obesity* study is this: The authors reported that their data *supported* the U.S. government guidelines of a goal of sixty minutes per day of moderate to vigorous physical activity.

Slaving away on a bike or treadmill to lose only four to six pounds (1.8 to 2.7 kg) a year . . . and that's a pro? It sounds like a con to us.

There's plenty more research that shows weight loss from cardio is meager. In mixed-gender studies, most of the success stories are men, raising the average weight loss. Other times, it's the obese individuals in the participant pool, who often initially shed weight more quickly than those who are less overweight.

Slaving away on a bike or treadmill to lose only four to six pounds (1.8 to 2.7 kg) a year . . . and that's a pro? It sounds like a con to us.

In a 2008 study from the *International Journal of Obesity*, British researchers led an exercise intervention with thirty-five overweight and obese men and women to see how much weight they could lose in twelve weeks.[29] Previously sedentary participants exercised five times a week for the duration of the study. They could choose from treadmills, stationary bikes, rowing machines, and step machines for their workouts.

After twelve weeks, participants lost an average of 8.2 pounds (3.7 kg). But a closer look reveals this: The people with the most weight to lose were skewing the average.

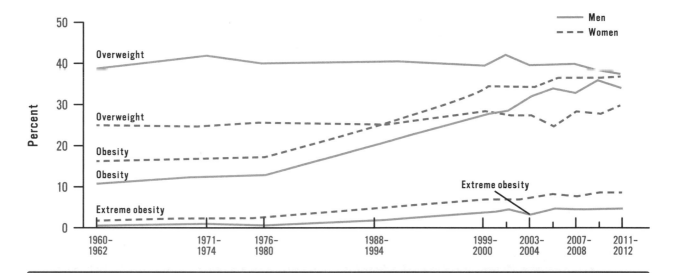

U.S. OVERWEIGHT AND OBESITY RATES[30]
Figure 1.2: Trends in U.S. overweight and obesity rates from 1960 to 2012

Only half the participants lost as much or more than predicted, and these tended to be the heaviest subjects. The other half of the group lost less than expected, and, in some cases, actually gained weight—stair-stepping five days a week and *gaining* weight.

So if you're lucky, you might be above the eight-pound (3.6 kg) weight loss mark after twelve weeks of cardio. But based on findings from studies like the one just noted, if you're a woman with just fifteen, thirty, or forty-five pounds (6.8, 13.6, or 20.4 kg) to lose, you have a better chance of stepping your way to weight *gain* with a regimen like this.

To be honest, I'm not even sure how the "weight loss from cardio" myth caught on. Aerobics was originally sold as a program for "health and longevity fitness." The promise: It

might help prevent a heart attack, and it will probably make you feel better.[31] Dr. Cooper didn't say the weight would start dropping off.

In fact, it's common for people to gain weight when training for a marathon—and not because they're gaining muscle weight.[32] (Stay tuned for more on this.)

Losing weight isn't just a vanity thing. As you'll see in the next chapter, shedding excess bodyweight—more specifically, body fat—is associated with a lower risk of type 2 diabetes and other metabolic disturbances, along with a host of other health benefits. So finding exercise that pairs with your diet to help you maintain a healthy bodyweight should, indeed, be the goal.

THE CLASSIC *JAMA* STUDY REVISITED

So what about heart health? Didn't the Cooper Institute's landmark 1989 study prove that aerobics was necessary to stave off disease and keep the cardiorespiratory system in good shape?

Dr. Cooper's team showed a relationship between reduced mortality and physical fitness. But was it proof of a relationship between longevity and *aerobics*?

The answer is no.

At least not according to the data published in the study. There was no mention of whether participants engaged in running, cycling, walking, or even *any* physical activity during the eight-year study period. Researchers simply recorded how well participants performed in the fitness test.

Evidence was compelling that the fitter participants were likely to live longer. But for all we know, they were lifting weights, doing sprints, playing sports, or even simply working a physically demanding job.

Yet, the study was hailed as proof the aerobics program worked.

Here's another mystery. The Cooper Institute's influential *JAMA* study included, as a basis for their inquiry, a prior study that found a correlation between longevity and exercise. This earlier study, published in 1975, found heart health benefits linked to work-related physical activity.[33]

That study observed longshoremen in the San Francisco Bay area, and was one of several groundbreaking studies in the 1960s and '70s that compared longshoremen and railroad workers to desk clerks, and found the first group dying less from coronary heart disease.[34]

What type of work activity were the longshoremen doing? Lifting and short bursts of intense exertion.

Yet, functional fitness, such as work-related physical activity, wasn't part of Cooper's exercise prescription. In fact, in his first book, he was fervently against weightlifting and interval training. He claimed in *Aerobics* that interval workouts delivered no health benefits and lifting was "unnatural."

It's unclear, then, what Cooper thought the longshoremen in the 1975 study—which he cited often in his own research—were doing to reap health benefits. It is unlikely these workers, in addition to loading and unloading ships all day, were penciling in a brisk thirty- to sixty-minute daily walk!

WHAT THE RESEARCH REALLY SAYS ABOUT WEIGHT LOSS AND EXERCISE

Decades of studies show negligible weight loss results from activities, such as walking and jogging, at moderate intensity. Other types of exercise, including high-intensity interval exercise and strength training, have emerged as superior for fat loss.[35]

Take the findings of one leading HIIE researcher, Dr. Stephen Boutcher, at the School of Medical Sciences at University of New South Wales, Australia. In a 2010 *Journal of Obesity* review of the previous fifteen years of research, Boutcher concluded the following:

1. High-intensity intermittent sprinting exercise appears to be more effective than other types of exercise at reducing subcutaneous and abdominal body fat.

2. HIIE results in significantly greater fat loss in women compared to steady-state exercise.

3. Regular HIIE significantly increases both aerobic and anaerobic fitness.[36]

As for strength training, the more muscle mass you have, the more calories your body burns. Thus, an exercise program that decreases fat mass while increasing muscle tissue (e.g., bodyweight circuits) helps achieve the lean body look and overall health you desire.

It's strange, then, that interval and strength workouts were marginalized with the cardio boom.

Strength exercises were fine to do on the side, Kenneth Cooper said in his book *Aerobics*. He even included "some basic calisthenics" in his routine. But overall, weightlifting was really only good for one thing, he wrote: weightlifting.

What's more, lifting could lead to injury and bulking up disproportionately, he cautioned. It also tended to fool people into thinking they were fitter than they really were. He had the same thing to say about interval workouts, or sprints: Why bother? Aerobics was the golden ticket to health and longevity; you might as well keep it safe and simple.

The anti-weightlifting, anti-sprint message Cooper preached wasn't grounded in research. His cardio-or-bust approach seemed, simply, to serve his own preference for running, a passion for which he was famous. Many other proponents of cardio revealed the same bias: They enjoyed it. They wanted it to be a panacea.

Of course, doing something you enjoy isn't inherently bad—and if it means you'll exercise regularly, that's a good thing. The problem is that a strong preference for cardio led many experts to say "the more, the merrier" (to the point of calling excessive aerobics a "positive addiction"[37]) and to ignore other avenues for exercise. Cooper didn't cite studies when he cast down strength and interval exercises in his books; in fact, he ignored the piles of research that established their effectiveness.

Perhaps most puzzlingly, the Cooper Institute doesn't seem to have tested weightlifting or sprints in comparison to aerobics—or at all.

WHY WAS FUNCTIONAL FITNESS IGNORED?

"By the 1970s, according to many economists, the man who works with his hands will be almost extinct," Kennedy lamented in his famous *Sports Illustrated* rallying cry. Is it odd that the types of physical activity encountered naturally prior to advancements in technology—lifting and sprinting in bursts of exertion, just like the longshoremen in the heart health study—were replaced with running, something that hasn't been part of our daily lives for thousands of years?

No one would deny Kenneth Cooper's tremendous impact on health and exercise habits. But even he doesn't believe what he said about cardio in the 1960s.

Cooper devoted his career to helping the world find ways to achieve vitality and well-being; aerobics was just his early theory to get us there. Since then, he, like many other cardio campaigners, has updated his prescription for fitness. As a researcher, he couldn't deny the studies that prove the value of strength and interval training. Nor could he deny his own experience—the aches and pains that cardio brought on as he got older. (See more about Cooper's change of heart in chapter 7.)

Now, he also says *more* cardio is not better. And he doesn't say, "run," he says, "exercise."

Yet, people haven't been getting the word. Even though Cooper has been spreading a new message since the 1990s, those early claims stuck.[38] Many are still thumbing through their tattered copies of the 1968 book. It was drilled into Americans' heads for so long: Cardio is good; weights are bad.

No one would deny Kenneth Cooper's tremendous impact on health and exercise habits. But even he doesn't believe what he said about cardio in the 1960s.

Those outdated notions linger that strength training leads to injury, is for body builders, and has no functional value outside the weight room.

A look back through the history of exercise turns up all kinds of erroneous, cultural-based guidelines. Remember when women weren't allowed to run marathons . . . in the *sixties*? Kathrine Switzer famously snuck into the Boston Marathon in 1967 just to prove that women could run all twenty-six miles (41.8 km) without fainting. After she crossed the finish line, marathon officials were forced to change their blatantly biased and completely irrational rule.

The idea about the "dangers" of strength training that took hold in the aerobics era wasn't much different.

In truth, people are not more likely to hurt themselves doing squats than running around a park. If you're not squatting properly, you might suffer some discomfort or an acute injury. But avid cardio exercisers are more likely to suffer the deeper, irreversible injuries over time (for the gory details, see chapter 5).

As for the claim that weightlifting is only good for weightlifting, perhaps Cooper never considered lifting a heavy box. Or pushing a lawnmower. Or chopping wood. Somewhere along the way it seems that weightlifting and muscular builds got associated with the lower classes, who were still working physically laborious jobs, while "skinny" became a sign of one's ability to spend hours swimming, playing tennis, riding a bike, and circling the suburban block in white sneakers every morning.

But try to pick up a heavy box when your only form of exercise is running and you'll *really* see what causes injury. If anything, it seems like the only exercise that has almost no practical, everyday application is . . . cardio.

THE WORST OFFENDER: GOVERNMENT GUIDELINES

Despite clear evidence (and advice from the father of aerobics himself) that *more* cardio is not better for weight loss or heart health, and that it can actually be harmful, government recommendations for cardiovascular activity have only shifted in one direction over the years—up.

Currently, the goal of the Healthy People 2020 initiative[39] is to have Americans doing more than 300 minutes per week of moderate aerobic activity or more than 150 minutes per week of vigorous aerobic activity. On the upper end of the guideline, that's 42 minutes a day, seven days a week—or 50 minutes a day, if you want a day off.

Sufficient, but less than ideal, would be at least 150 minutes a week of moderate aerobic activity or 75 minutes a week of vigorous aerobic activity, they suggest.

As for strength training, it's an "extra." You should do it, they say, but they don't give specific guidelines. There's no mention at all of alternatives, such as interval workouts or sprints. If one were to substitute "vigorous aerobic activity" for high-intensity interval workouts, then even 75 minutes per week would be sufficient (and 150 minutes would probably be too much).

Once again, steady-state cardio is misrepresented as the golden standard of exercise, in amounts that aren't feasible for most people.

Popular online health resources, such as the Mayo Clinic and WebMD, simply repeat these guidelines.[40] Sadly, this is where the majority of the public gets exercise information. Even those who ask their doctors are likely to get the same advice: Take a 60-minute walk every day. Only those who can afford to hire a personal trainer, or who know which books and magazines to turn to, have been lucky enough to get the real story about what is effective for fat loss and health . . . until now.

A NEW PROMISE

Remember Catherine? Instead of trying to convince her that she needed to drop her cardio regimen, I decided to *show* her—with a program of interval training and body-weight circuits like the ones in this book. She also adopted a sensible diet, similar to what you'll find in chapter 9. Twelve weeks later, Catherine was down 14 pounds (6.4 kg), had trimmed 6 inches (15 cm) off her waist, and in place of dimpled arms and thighs was a toned, muscular figure.

For most people, the runaway cardio guidelines have either led to a hate relationship with exercise or they've become an excuse to do nothing at all. An estimated 80 percent of

Catherine, before and after three rounds of twelve-week interval and strength-training regimens.

Americans don't get the ideal amount of physical activity. It's a shame, since there have been better, faster, proven alternatives all along.

It's time for doctors, health advisers, and journalists to take a closer look and admit the evidence isn't there. Exercise scientists must stop trying to package meager results from their studies as "support" for outdated guidelines. Journalists must get diligent about reading past the study abstracts, or worse, only skimming the press releases, which leads to spreading exaggerated results far and wide.

For most people, the runaway cardio guidelines have either led to a hate relationship with exercise or they've become an excuse to do nothing at all. An estimated 80 percent of Americans don't get the ideal amount of physical activity. It's a shame, since there have been better, faster, proven alternatives all along.

Above all, government organizations leading national exercise campaigns must open their eyes to the current research, which suggests that excessive cardio is not only ineffective and unrealistic for most people, but it can be dangerous. In addition to contributing to the retention of harmful body fat and the reduction of muscle mass—both of which *increase* one's risk of disease—endurance exercise has the potential to put excessive strain on the heart and the joints.

Other forms of exercise, such as strength training and "sprint" workouts, can produce better weight-loss results, along with cardiovascular benefits. Numerous studies have also shown that these forms of exercise can boost your mood and enhance psychological well-being.[41] And without a doubt, strength and short burst workouts rival cardio in delivering stress relief, exercise endorphins, and—ahem—a better sex life.

WHAT YOU NEED TO KNOW

- Despite constantly increasing rates of aerobic exercise over the past forty years, the percentage of overweight adults has remained fairly constant and obesity rates have risen dramatically.

- Seminal research showing a link between exercise and reduced risk of coronary heart disease was not looking at aerobic exercise specifically. In fact, most data pertained to work-related physical activity, which most likely included heavy lifting and bursts of exertion, closer to an interval cardio and strength-training regimen!

- National exercise guidelines are due for an update. At best, endurance cardio is obsolete compared to today's training methods. At worst, it's ineffective and unfeasible for most Americans, and too much can cause harm (see chapter 5).

- Dr. Kenneth Cooper, the father of aerobics, changed his mind about cardio. His message went from, "there's no such thing as too much" to, "cardio in moderation," to, ultimately, "cardio is part of a balanced approach that should include strength exercises." Here's what the message *should* be: cardio is optional, but be aware of the risks—and don't rely on it for long-term weight loss.

50% of Americans log 150 minutes of cardio a week.

68.7% of Americans are overweight.

2

THE WEIGHT LOSS SCAM

IMAGINE THIS. IT'S ANOTHER busy day at work. Your kids are hungry. The fridge is bare. No one else is going to make dinner. It's up to you again.

You rush from your desk to the grocery store and then drive home through the beginning of rush-hour traffic. Chicken fingers and fries get put on the table, and you eat too much of them cleaning up the kids' plates. Now you're supposed to brave the end of rush-hour traffic and drive back across town for a 6:30 p.m. aerobics class. Either that or go for a forty-five-minute run around the neighborhood—through the same nightmarish traffic.

The anxiety that comes with the thought of sitting in your car crawling through traffic (or choking on car exhaust jogging through it), plus the post-dinner carbohydrate coma from those tasty fries, sap all your willpower. It's off to the couch again—same as last night. Tomorrow is unlikely to be different.

And that, ladies and gentlemen of the jury, is why cardio is guilty of killing your motivation. It's not a practical exercise solution for most people. Even if you did manage to spend the one to two hours from door to door, it probably wouldn't be worth it, as you've surely learned the hard way. This was the story of my mom's life and why she was never able to make cardio a habit.

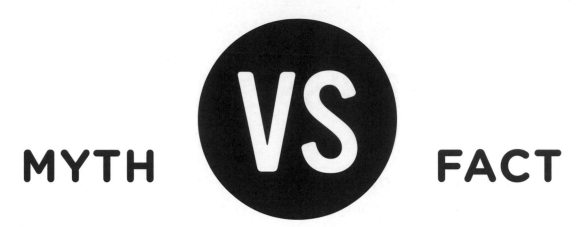

MYTH VS FACT

MYTH	FACT
Aerobic exercise is the best kind for fat loss.	Mounting research shows that high-intensity interval exercise reduces fat faster.
Strength training isn't going to help someone lose weight.	Strength training promotes fat loss by increasing your muscle mass and, thus, metabolism. The more muscle you have, the more calories you'll burn during exercise *and* rest!
If you burn more calories during a cardio workout than HIIT or strength training, that proves it's better for fat loss.	There's much more to exercise-induced fat loss than the number of calories burned during a workout.
There's no harm in having a little excess body fat.	Excess fat, especially deep belly fat, can pose a serious health risk—it has been linked with heart disease, diabetes, and other major conditions.

But unfeasible exercise plans are killing more than motivation. We can joke about middle-age spread, but having a stomach roll over your jeans isn't just a matter of looks—excess body fat and a couch-potato lifestyle are poised to overtake smoking as the leading cause of preventable death in the United States and worldwide.[42]

Globally, 3.2 million people die every year from complications of being overweight and out of shape.[43] This deadly combo is linked with increased risk for heart disease, type 2 diabetes, and many types of cancer.[44]

What's the harm? First, as with dietary fat, not all body fat is created equal. There are two kinds: subcutaneous fat, which is above the muscle, and visceral fat, which is the round, hard belly fat underneath the stomach muscle. It's visceral fat that delivers the death knell.

Globally, 3.2 million people die every year from complications of being overweight and out of shape.[43] This deadly combo is linked with increased risk for heart disease, type 2 diabetes, and many types of cancer.[44]

Doctors refer to this deep, abdominal fat as toxic fat because it releases a wide variety of harmful compounds in the blood associated with the previously mentioned diseases, leading us to an early grave (see Body Fat 101, page 39).[45]

For decades, ever since America moved from a manual labor workforce to a sedentary lifestyle, we've been looking for the best way to eliminate dangerous and unsightly body fat.[46] But these efforts have been no match for the widespread increase in caloric intake.

In 2000, the average American consumed 530 more calories than the average person in 1970, according to the United States Department of Agriculture (USDA).[47] The typical American diet had grown by an incredible 25 percent.

In addition to diet, we know that sleep quality, stress level, and genetics play a role in our ability to regulate bodyweight.[48-49] Nonetheless, physical activity can, and should, be a part of everyone's lifelong plan to fight fat. The right exercise can help prevent the accumulation of both kinds of body fat—including that deadly deep belly fat—as well as provide myriad other health benefits, as we'll discuss in later chapters.

All this is to say, yes, you should be exercising for fat loss. Yes, it can help prolong your life. And, yes, the *type* of exercise matters.

CARDIO VERSUS INTERVAL EXERCISE: INTENSITY IS KEY

I grew up hearing the same advice about aerobic activity as so many others. It was what people had to do when they wanted to get in shape. But at twenty-one, I tested it out for myself.

As I mentioned in the book's introduction, as a young college student gearing up for another summer soccer season, I set aside my usual strength-training routine for a high-volume cardio regimen, running thirty-plus miles (48 km) per week. Over those months, I got smaller and weaker; my muscles actually seemed to be shrinking, and I was getting slower on the field. By the end of summer, I gave up and switched back to my original fitness regimen of less—but more intense—exercise. Soon, I was stronger and fitter. Lesson learned!

The more I looked into it, the more I couldn't ignore the overwhelming evidence about steady-state cardio—and I wasn't the only one. After reviewing the body of studies conducted, Dr. Stephen Boutcher, one of the world's leading exercise researchers, wrote:

> *Most exercise protocols designed to induce fat loss have focused on regular steady-state exercise, such as walking and jogging, at a moderate intensity. Disappointingly, these kinds of protocols have led to negligible weight loss.*[50]

Disappointing indeed. But, as Boutcher and many other exercise scientists discovered, there *are* exercises that facilitate fat loss: high intensity interval exercise and strength training.

In fact, since the early 1990s, hundreds of researchers have published peer-reviewed evidence showing that people who do interval and resistance exercises come out slimmer than their cardio counterparts. Let's look at a few of the studies.

Exercise scientists discovered there are *exercises that facilitate fat loss: high intensity interval exercise and strength training.*

Angelo Tremblay, Ph.D., is a pioneering researcher on obesity and energy balance and lead author of the first study on high-intensity exercise for fat loss. At the time of this study, in 1994, Tremblay was affiliated with a group of scientists in the Physical Activity Sciences Laboratory at Laval University in Quebec. They were intrigued by a large dataset, which they'd published in 1990, revealing that subjects who exercised at a higher intensity were leaner than lower-intensity exercisers despite energy expenditure, or calorie burn, being equal.[51]

With data on 1,366 females and 1,257 males, Tremblay and his team had reason to believe that continuous, low- to moderate-intensity exercise might not be the gold standard for weight loss after all.

That's strange. According to popular wisdom around the superiority of the so-called

ENDURANCE TRAINING GROUP
Program time: 20 weeks
Total number of workouts: 80
Ultimate time per workout: 45 minutes
Mean estimated energy expenditure: 120.4 MJ

30 min   45 min

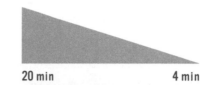

HIIE GROUP
Program time: 15 weeks
Total number of workouts: 60
Ultimate time per workout: 4 minutes
Mean estimated energy expenditure: 57.9 MJ

20 min   4 min

ENDURANCE TRAINING VERSUS HIIE STUDY RESULTS
Figure 2.1: Battling the bulge: Despite significantly shorter workouts and a shorter program duration, participants in the high-intensity interval group fared better than the exercisers in Dr. Tremblay and colleagues' 1994 study—they dropped nine times the subcutaneous fat for a given energy expenditure.

fat-burning zone, which is supposedly reached after twenty minutes of low to moderate cardio exertion, shouldn't the results have been the other way around?

To solve the mystery, they gathered twenty-seven men and women, designed a training program, and divided participants between two exercise conditions.[52]

Group 1 was the endurance training (ET) group. These participants cycled at a continuous pace, starting at thirty minutes per session, and progressing to forty-five minutes. They logged a total of eighty workouts during a twenty-week training period.

Group 2 did short, high-intensity interval exercise (HIIE). They started with a few weeks of thirty-minute steady-state cycling for conditioning, but, by week 5, this was phased out and participants were doing short interval workouts of roughly four minutes. The HIIE program was shorter, lasting only fifteen weeks for a total of sixty workouts.

At the end of the study, Tremblay's team gathered the outcome data, and sure enough, participants in the interval workout group (Group 2) lost more fat than those in the cardio group. This was true even though people in the HIIE condition did twenty fewer workouts and exercised for a shorter duration each time.

Now, participants' weight didn't budge in either group. But their body fat did. The average decrease in subcutaneous skin fat, measured by a skinfold caliper, was *nine times greater* in the HIIE program.

Basically, the participants had dropped fat pounds and gained muscle weight in its place.

Not only did these interval exercisers lose more body fat, they also improved their muscle metabolism more than the steady cyclers. Most interesting of all: Exercise-induced energy expenditure in the HIIE program was *half* that of the ET program.

That's an important distinction. Energy expenditure is essentially the same thing as calorie burn. We have resting energy expenditure (the basal metabolic rate) and energy expenditure during exercise. I'll explain this further in chapter 4, but it's vital to note the difference because it shows us how the impact of a workout goes beyond calorie burn *during* the workout. If a workout helps you build muscle, then you're going to increase muscle mass and burn more fat in the end.

All in all, the interval exercisers got much more bang for their exercise buck.

This groundbreaking study was the first of many of its kind and hinted at some of the mechanisms that would lead people to lose more fat from interval exercise than steady-state exercise.

It all flew in the face of what experts were telling us, and, as a young graduate student finishing my degree in exercise science, I couldn't wait to learn more. Obviously, the popular health belief that "more is better for weight loss" was completely wrong.

I also had my own anecdotal evidence in hand. During my studies, I was sequestered in the biochemistry lab from morning until night, and I only had time for a thirty-minute trip to the gym. But by applying what I knew about strength and interval training, these short, intense workouts had me in the best shape of my life!

Research on HIIT continued to emerge throughout the 1990s, such as that from Japanese researcher Izumi Tabata, who tested four-minute HIIT workouts against lengthy cardio sessions. The four-minute sprinting workout proved superior for fitness gains and would later become known as the popular Tabata Protocol, which is covered in chapter 4.

Obviously, the popular health belief that "more is better for weight loss" was completely wrong.

Although Dr. Tabata's HIIT program required maximum intensity, the workouts tested in other HIIT studies did not. Studies continued to show that exercise intensity didn't need to be vomit inducing for people to achieve superior fat loss. It just needed to be, for short durations, more intense than the typical continuous-pace bike ride or jog through the park.

REPLICATING THE HIIT RESULTS

Following in the footsteps of Tremblay's research team, numerous exercise physiology labs around the world have tested HIIT against cardio and come to the same conclusion.[53]

One such experiment, led by Dr. Ethlyn Trapp and a team of Australian researchers (including Dr. Boutcher), compared HIIT to steady-state exercise in young, sedentary women.[54] The 2008 study didn't require the interval exercisers to push themselves to their physical limit. Instead, women alternated between eight seconds of sprinting and twelve seconds of slow pedaling, working their way up from five-minute workouts to twenty minutes by the end of the program.

Meanwhile, women in the steady-state exercise (SSE) program cycled at a continuous moderate intensity, starting with ten to twenty minutes and working their way up to forty-minute sessions. The third control group did no exercise.

Once again, participants fared better in the HIIT group. After fifteen weeks of exercising three times per week, only the HIIT group had significant fat loss, with notable reductions in fat around their torsos and legs. These women lost an average of 5.5 pounds (2.5 kg) of overall body fat mass.

While the HIIT group got great results, the SSE group had *gained* a pound (0.5 kg) of fat by the end of the program. That's right—gained. The cardio exercisers increased fat mass slightly more than the control group, who did no exercise at all.

The study authors concluded that individuals are likely to get better fat loss results from high-intensity interval exercise in twenty minutes a day, three times a week, compared with three, forty-minute cardio workouts a week.

A similar experiment by researchers at the University of Virginia found the same thing. Obese middle-aged women in an HIIT program lost significantly more abdominal fat—both visceral and subcutaneous—than women in a low-intensity aerobics program.[55] In fact, the low-intensity exercise group lost as much fat as the control group—none. (But hey, at least they didn't *gain* a pound [0.5 kg]!)

AN UPLIFTING ALTERNATIVE: STRENGTH TRAINING

Are you hoping to get off that bike altogether? No problem. Although short burst workouts can be done with cardio activities, such as cycling, as in the studies discussed previously, an HIIT workout can also use bodyweight resistance exercises: For example, doing burpees (or squat thrusts) for twenty seconds, followed by ten seconds of rest, then jumping jacks, rest, mountain climbers, rest, and so on for eight rounds (four minutes total).

Whether you're doing an HIIT workout with resistance exercise or doing push-ups and squats at your normal pace, research has shown that strength training can trump cardio for fat loss benefits.

It brings us right back to what we know about physiology: Lean muscle mass is associated with higher resting metabolism, or how many calories you burn when you're not exercising. Strength training increases muscle, whereas aerobic training does not (and sometimes actually reduces it).

One of the earliest studies to report this phenomenon was conducted by a group of researchers at West Virginia University in 1999.[56] They compared aerobic training to resistance training, each in combination with a diet.

In this study, resting metabolism decreased in the cardio group, and they lost both weight *and* lean muscle mass. Muscle loss (catabolism) is exacerbated by calorie restriction. Only the strength training group was able to lose weight without losing muscle mass or experiencing a reduction in resting metabolic rate.

Whether you're doing an HIIT workout with resistance exercise or doing push-ups and squats at your normal pace, research has shown that strength training can trump cardio for fat loss benefits.

Another study, this one led by a team of Korean researchers, compared aerobics training with a combined aerobics-and-strength-training program.[57] Participants in the sample were obese, middle-aged women. One-third of participants did aerobics (we're talking the 1980s kind: grapevines, rock steps, and cha-cha-chas), while one-third replaced 50 percent of their workouts with resistance training. The final third, a control group, didn't exercise.

After six months, the group that incorporated strength training was cha-cha-cha-ing for joy: They had significant reductions in visceral and subcutaneous fat, above and beyond the aerobics-only group. The combined exercise group was also the only group to see significant gains in lean muscle.

While the combined aerobics-and-resistance routine was clearly effective for fat loss, there was a downside to the program design: Women in both exercise conditions were working out six days a week, for one hour each time. That's an extreme time commitment that few people could pull off in real life.

Not to worry. With a more efficient program design, you can spend less time than these women did and still get the same or *better* improvements in body composition.

The one-hour aerobics workout? Replace it with a short HIIT workout. The one-hour resistance training session? I have no idea what they were doing for that much time! But I do know they used strength exercises that worked only a small amount of muscle mass, such as leg raises, abdominal crunches, and barbell curls. That's an outmoded form of training, and compound movements like the ones I'll show you in this book, which work multiple large muscle groups at once, are much more efficient for increasing lean muscle and shedding fat . . . in a fraction of the time.

BODY FAT 101

Is body fat all bad and how do we measure it, anyway?

Body Composition
Weight doesn't tell the whole story. Often we use the term "weight loss" because it's what people know, but what we really care about is improvement in body composition—that is, a decrease in excess body fat and/or an increase in muscle. Muscle is more dense than fat, which is why you can get slimmer and more toned without losing weight. It's also why most exercise studies (should) report changes in body fat mass and inches, not just weight.

Body Mass Index (BMI)
This is a ratio of height to weight. While not an accurate indicator of body fat percentage, a strong correlation exists between body fat and BMI—unless you have above-average amounts of muscle.[58] A BMI of 18.5 to 24.9 is considered healthy; 25 to 29.9 is overweight; and 30 or higher is obese.

Disease Risk
The medical field generally agrees that excess body fat raises a person's risk of health trouble. Mortality increases in BMIs of 25 and up; the incline becomes more dramatic in BMIs over 30.[59] In one study, participants with a BMI of 35 or higher were twice as likely to develop heart disease or stroke, 1.5 times more likely to develop colon cancer, and more than twice as likely to develop hypertension and gall stones[60]—and twenty (20!) times more likely to develop diabetes.

Visceral Fat (the Harmful Belly Fat)
Medical experts believe we should be most worried about deep abdominal fat—fat below the stomach muscles—thought to be particularly toxic due to its proximity to the portal vein that sends blood from the intestinal area to the liver.[61] Visceral fat releases biochemicals into the blood that can increase insulin resistance and negatively impact blood pressure, blood clotting, and cholesterol levels.[62] Experts believe exercise is one of the best ways to reduce visceral fat.[63]

THE PROBLEM WITH CARDIO STUDIES

The majority of health organizations in America continue to recommend one hour of cardio per day for weight maintenance.[64-65] Some guidelines cite scientific evidence, but that evidence deserves a closer look.

Recall the 2007 *Obesity* study from chapter 1 (see page 22), where researchers cried "weight loss!" from sixty minutes of moderate to vigorous cardio six days a week.[66] But the results were disappointing. In one year, men in the study lost an average of around 6.5 pounds (2.9 kg) of fat, and female participants lost just 4 pounds (1.8 kg).

Three hundred hours of cardio couldn't help these previously sedentary people whittle more than a few centimeters off their waists. And the poor folks who did anything fewer than thirty minutes a day saw no fat loss from cardio whatsoever.

Participants seemed to fare better in a 2008 study from the University of Leeds. Here, sedentary men and women subjects lost, on average, 8.2 pounds (3.7 kg) of bodyweight in twelve weeks from a five-times-a-week cardio regimen.[67]

Yet, some unlucky participants, once again, gained weight from body fat. Can you imagine? Standing in front of a mirror after logging sixty sweat-drenched workouts on a treadmill or stair-stepper, only to observe . . . you're *wider* than before?

It is studies like these that "support" the current federal recommendations for aerobic exercise. Why do these studies give us misleading results? First, the body's response to exercise is influenced by a person's sex, as well as age and starting weight. Why is that important? Because many studies showing fat loss from cardio have failed to differentiate between groups when reporting results.[68]

More often than not, it's *men* who lost a few pounds, bringing up the average (sorry ladies).[69-70] Time for the cold-hard truth about cardio: Women are even *less* likely to lose weight from steady-state exercise than men.[71]

This is ironic, since "weight loss" wasn't advertised as a major benefit of cardio until Dr. Cooper and others began extending their exercise advice to women (and dance aerobics was born).

Women may have a harder time losing weight in any exercise regimen because men typically have more muscle and less body fat—in part due to the hormone testosterone—and this affects metabolism. But another reason could be differences in food preferences or calorie consumption.[72] As you'll see in chapter 6, women tend to be more susceptible to calorie and carb increases in response to cardio.

Here's another reason some people get confused about cardio and fat loss: The more fat you have to lose, the faster you'll lose it, no matter what exercise you're doing. Just think of the contestants on *The Biggest Loser*—at the beginning of the competition their weight loss is dramatic.

This is why individuals who are very overweight or obese may successfully reduce body fat with cardio at first, only to be confused when they can't shake that last forty or sixty pounds (18 or 27 kg). *Cardio was working before*, they think. *Maybe I just need to do MORE.*

Even when researchers do divulge the caveats of their positive cardio results, or when they tell us the results may only apply to a specific subset of the population, it doesn't seem to stop the results from being generalized in recommendations.

We should mention that the interval and strength training research in this chapter found successful fat loss and lean muscle gain across age groups, for men and women, and for people ranging from slender to obese. Put simply, these seem to hold up in scientific trials as the best ways to improve your body composition, no matter who you are.

HOW THE FOCUS ON "WEIGHT" MISLEADS US

Some cardio studies do find significant "weight loss" from aerobic exercise, and a whole lot of cardio fans can say they've watched the numbers go down on the scale. But, as we've learned, it's sometimes for the wrong reason: muscle loss. Let's talk more about the role of muscle for a minute.

Looking back to the 1990 data published by Dr. Tremblay and his colleagues, bodyweight didn't differ much between the higher-intensity and lower-intensity exercisers. But

both men and women in the higher-intensity group had narrower waist circumference and a healthier waist-to-hip ratio—two correlates of the amount of visceral adipose tissue.

It's not uncommon for walkers and runners to become "skinny fat." That's when muscle atrophies, or shrinks, rendering the body smaller but weak and flabby.

In their subsequent 1994 study, bodyweight stayed the same for participants in both the HIIT and the endurance training programs. But the HIIT group lost fat and inches, while the steady-state cardio group did not. It's not uncommon for walkers and runners to become "skinny fat." That's when muscle atrophies, or shrinks, rendering the body smaller but weak and flabby.

Here's the scientific explanation. Long cardio workouts sometimes catabolize (break down) amino acids to use for fuel in the energy-producing reactions needed in cardio. This takes place during long sessions—greater than thirty minutes—and happens even faster if a person is in caloric restriction. When this happens, the amino acids required for fuel come from a breakdown in nonworking muscle tissue and are released from muscle cells to go to the liver. In the liver, the nitrogen is removed and the carbon skeleton of the amino acids is shuttled into the working muscles.

Picture a cyclist with tiny arms. Working muscles (legs) use energy from catabolized muscle (arms).

Building muscle (anabolism) can have the opposite effect than cardio exercise because the body uses fat to fuel muscle growth. Amino acids are the "bricks" of muscle building, and the process requires energy that must come from stored carbohydrate or stored fat.

Lean muscle mass also makes a significant contribution to your basal metabolic rate, or BMR. This describes the rate at which your body burns calories at rest.

Now, the common belief that a pound (0.5 kg) of muscle burns fifty calories is, sadly, just a myth (if only). But it is true that muscle uses more calories at rest than fat.[73] That's one reason resistance exercise helps reduce body fat, regardless of how much you burn during the actual workout. It's also why cardio can take a slow, creeping toll on your body composition over time, no matter how much energy you expend during a cardio session—which, as you'll see in part 2, is probably a lot less than you think.

Now seems like a good time to reinforce one point: The number of calories burned during a workout is only a small part of the fat loss picture. The calories-in, calories-out equation just isn't that simple. Jogging for an hour may indeed (sometimes) burn more calories than a typical HIIT or strength-training workout. But don't slap on your pedometer just yet.

First, you must consider the "afterburn." Also known as excess post-exercise oxygen consumption, or EPOC, the afterburn effect basically means you burn more calories for a longer period of time after your workout. It is associated with intense exercise, both interval training and resistance training, and you'll learn more about it in chapter 4.

There's yet another important factor in fat loss that needs mentioning. That is how well your sweat sessions help you regulate insulin. Research indicates that an ongoing HIIT regimen can do more to reduce or prevent insulin resistance than steady-state cardio.[74] Although we'll explain metabolic syndrome in detail in chapter 7, for now, just know that lower fasting insulin levels reveal a better metabolic profile; essentially, if you are lean and fit, your fasting insulin will be low . . . if you're fat and prediabetic, your insulin will be high. As you'll see in the next chapter, higher body fat, especially belly fat, increases your risk of diabetes, as well as heart disease and stroke.

KEEP SOME CARDIO, JUST NOT FOR FAT LOSS

If all this has you scratching your head about why cardio is still heavily recommended for fat loss and ultimate health, join the club. Here's a telling figure: Approximately 50 percent of Americans have met the federal guideline for aerobic activity since 2009.[75] Yet, 68.7 percent of the adult population is overweight. How is it that half the people in the United States are logging more than 150 minutes of weekly moderate-intensity cardio, yet two-thirds are in the unhealthy weight range?

Obviously, aerobic activity is not the answer we need. In fact, it's kind of like trying to pay off a loan by borrowing more money at a higher interest rate.

With regard to fat loss, science has shown that steady-state cardio is less effective than other exercises because it only burns energy *during* the workout, and when it doesn't incorporate resistance—as is the case with most cardio—it can decrease lean muscle mass. As you'll discover in the coming chapters, there are a slew of secondary reasons why steady-state cardio can halt fat loss. Instead of questioning its efficacy, most health officials have guessed that if it's not working, the solution is to do *more*. This mentality had *Biggest Loser* contestants exercising nine hours a week to maintain their results from the show, at the recommendation of the TV program's doctor. One contestant bleakly referred to it as a "life sentence."

How is it that half the people in the United States are logging more than 150 minutes of weekly moderate-intensity cardio, yet two-thirds are in the unhealthy weight range?

Let's be clear on one thing: It's not that cardio has *no* health benefits. It's that many of the touted benefits aren't there.

If you enjoy cardio, then, certainly, include it in your exercise regimen. I use low-intensity activities, such as walking my dog, to stay active for thirty minutes on rest days. Some of my clients dance, play sports, ride bikes, chase their children, or hike on "off" days, and these will certainly add to your health rewards.

But if your goal is fat loss, you don't need to spend hours a week on cardio to achieve it. In fact, fleeing the treadmill might be the best thing you do for your waistline.

WHAT YOU NEED TO KNOW

- Traditional steady-state cardio is not an efficient way to lose weight, especially for women and individuals who are only moderately overweight.

- Weight loss in the early stages of an aerobic training regimen can be misleading: You may be losing water weight and pounds of precious muscle, not belly fat.

- Combining cardio with a very-low-calorie diet is the *worst* way to try to shed fat because it can increase muscle loss and, in turn, lower metabolism.

Death rates are higher among people who jog 4 or more times per week than people who don't jog at all.

3

WHY CARDIO WON'T MAKE YOU LIVE LONGER

" **S**OME THIRTY MILLION Americans are running religiously, to save their lives—in essence, the quality of life itself," one aerobics book proclaimed in 1981.[76]

And this claim that we could stockpile immunity continued until running icons started dropping dead at shockingly young ages. American running legend Jim Fixx was among them.

Fixx set out on a run one day in 1984 while visiting the town of Hardwick, Vermont. His body was discovered on the side of the road, clad only in shorts and sneakers. He had died of a heart attack. Fixx was just fifty-two when he died. The cause of sudden death: coronary arteries damaged by arteriosclerosis. One artery was almost completely blocked.

Claims about runners' invincible hearts came under scrutiny after Fixx's shocking death and were ultimately disproven. Sadly, Fixx's death wasn't the last of them.

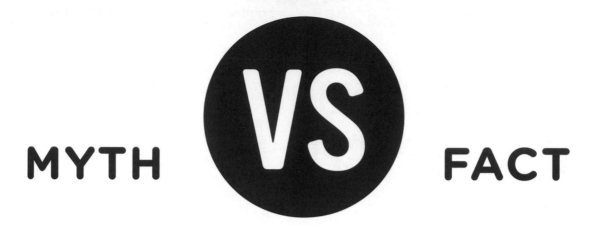

MYTH VS FACT

MYTH	FACT
Consistent cardio exercise guarantees longer life and a healthier heart.	Exercise can offer bonus heart protection, but it takes a backseat to several other major predictors of cardiovascular risk.
Cardio exercise is a license to eat poorly, smoke, or drink excessive amounts of alcohol.	Again, endurance is not life insurance.
Only cardio delivers cardiovascular benefits.	The heart health benefits observed in studies are not specific to cardio—they can be achieved with strengthening exercises and high-intensity interval training.
The relationship between exercise and health benefits is linear—the more exercise, the better for health.	While some exercise is vastly better than none, there is a U-shaped relationship between exercise and benefits: Past a certain threshold, the benefits begin to decline.

Brian Maxwell, the creator of the PowerBar, once ranked as the third-best marathoner in the world. He died of a heart attack at fifty-one.

Micah True, an American ultrarunner and mythic figure in Chris McDougall's book *Born to Run*, died unexpectedly of cardiac arrhythmia while running on a trail in New Mexico. He was fifty-eight.

At thirty-one, Miles Frost, the son of famed British broadcaster Sir David Frost, collapsed while jogging.[77] The avid jogger had a silent congenital heart condition. His death made big news in the U.K. in 2015—just two years after his father had died from a heart attack.

What caused all of these runners' hearts to stop suddenly, in many cases *mid run*? Some have argued that proper aerobic training is needed to prevent sudden cardiac death. But that wasn't the case here; these athletes were seasoned marathoners.

It is possible that the long, strenuous bouts of exercise actually led to heart damage or exacerbated an existing heart condition. There's ample evidence to suggest it can happen, as you'll see. But the bigger danger seems to be that they all bought into the same myth, that running would shield them from harm.

It's heartbreaking stories like these, along with others about forty-year-old men dying while running marathons, that forced me to speak up about the misguided cult adoration of cardio.

Most people, especially those who do cardio, go through the five stages of grief when I try to explain to them that cardio isn't a guarantee of a long life. First, they go through denial. Many of my clients are shocked to think of all the time they've wasted doing cardio, and they have a hard time accepting that their sense of being virtuous—as they trudged through countless hours of boredom and discomfort—was without merit.

Second, they respond with anger, and some clients, friends, and family members even accuse me of lying.

Third, they bargain to keep doing a little cardio outside of my programs, fanatically believing it still works.

Life not only goes on without cardio, but it goes on better, and with more time to focus on what really matters.

Fourth, depression sets in as they reminisce about hours spent lurched over a stairstepper or pounding on a treadmill without the benefits they so strongly believed in and thinking about what they could have done with that time.

Fifth, they reach a point of acceptance, usually after a week or two of doing my short burst workouts. Eventually, they realize that life not only goes on without cardio, but it goes on better, and with more time to focus on what really matters.

With any luck, I can usher you straight past these stages with a brief tour of the evidence.

We'll look at where the "aerobics is life insurance" promise began. And even further back, before the invention of aerobics, to where longevity benefits first made an appearance in the research—studies of occupational physical activity. Don't worry: There *is* good news at the end.

MEN AT WORK

It was the early 1950s, and epidemiologists had recently spotted a peculiar discrepancy among British social classes. Data revealed that men in higher social classes—professionals and businessmen—were dying from coronary heart disease at *twice* the rate of unskilled workers.[78] One group of medical researchers wondered if it had to do with the nature of the work; specifically, how much physical labor each group performed on the job. While much of society had moved into sedentary occupations, some jobs were still physically demanding.

To test their theory, Dr. Jerry Morris and his colleagues examined death rates among a large group of London bus drivers and bus conductors, the latter presumed to be more physically active. The results of the analysis were unveiled in *The Lancet*, a prestigious British medical journal, in 1953.[79] Sure enough, they found that fewer conductors were dying in middle age from coronary heart disease, compared with the stuck-on-their-rump bus drivers.

Related studies found a similar mortality rate gap between desk-bound postal clerks in London and Washington, D.C., and the postmen out delivering the mail.[80]

Throughout the 1950s and '60s, studies continued to find a relationship between sedentary jobs and fatal cardiovascular events. The active workers on small farms were suffering less coronary heart disease than managerial workers on large farms; and farmers had healthier hearts than men in less active occupations.[81]

In 1975, the *New England Journal of Medicine* published a twenty-two-year population study showing the same trend among longshoremen in California.[82] Over 6,000 men were ranked by level of exertion based on their job duties. Men who loaded and unloaded cargo were in the highly active category, while administrative workers were in the low activity category.

The data, yet again, suggested a protective effect from physical activity. The more active men had significantly fewer coronary deaths than the less-active jobholders, and cases of sudden cardiac death, in particular, were much less common for the "heavy workers." Notably, the death rates were not much different between the moderate and light activity workers.

All the research was pointing to *some* sort of connection between vigorous physical activity and heart health. But . . . what was it?

Epidemiologists couldn't say, exactly. Adding to the uncertainty, there was no way to say whether the effect was *causal*.

EXERCISE VERSUS PHYSICAL ACTIVITY

One key distinction in the research is that studies looking at "physical activity" include all kinds of movement throughout the day, including exercise, plus everything from yard work to climbing stairs to carrying groceries into the house.

"Exercise" specifically refers to structured physical activity, such as a workout routine.

The research has shown that both types of daily movement are beneficial. If you are highly active throughout the day and do weight-bearing activities that work all major muscle groups, you may not need to do structured exercise. However, there are important benefits to regimented workouts like the ones in this book:

- They enable you to meet specific health and fitness goals efficiently.

- You can track your time, intensity level, and progress. (It's easy to overestimate the time or exertion level you use in daily physical activity.)

My exercise goal is to spend *less* time by doing the *right* activities. This is how I ensure I'm meeting my health and fitness goals. That said, I recommend staying active in some form every day.

Observational studies can only show that a relationship exists somewhere among the variables. Maybe physical activity had a direct impact on cardiovascular risks—or maybe there was another factor in the mix. These groundbreaking studies all concluded on the same note: more research was needed.

This "proceed with caution" message got lost with the emergence of the aerobics movement in the 1960s. Coronary heart disease had been rising rapidly since the turn of the century, and the idea that we might have a cure—one as simple as a daily jog, no less—was mighty appealing.

Eager to spread the "good news," promoters of aerobic exercise took the early research and—forgive the pun—ran with it. Soon "physical activity" became "aerobics," and aerobic exercise became a "surefire" way to prevent heart disease. The more, the better, we were told.

What the public didn't see is this: The *type* of physical activity wasn't reported in most of these surveys, and when it was, it wasn't always aerobic exercise.

THE MYTH: EXERCISE GRANTS IMMUNITY

Participation in daily exercise reportedly doubled between 1961 and 1977. [86] It was hailed as a "fitness renaissance" as Americans took up swimming, bicycling, playing tennis, or the country's trendiest form of exercise— running—to buy extra years of life.

Early advocates of aerobics painted a pretty picture: Do a moderate amount of running, swimming, or cycling every week and you're in good shape; do a high amount and you're practically invincible.

The clan of running doctors who stood behind this message burgeoned in the 1970s and 80s. Cardiologists, such as Kenneth Cooper and George Sheehan, penned numerous bestselling guides to running and aerobics, including *Aerobics* and *Running and Being: The Total Experience*.

Dr. Thomas Bassler, a California physician and member of the American Medical Joggers Association, rose to acclaim with a 1977 journal article that declared more good news: an association between marathon running and immunity to atherosclerosis. [87] If you could run a marathon in under four hours, you

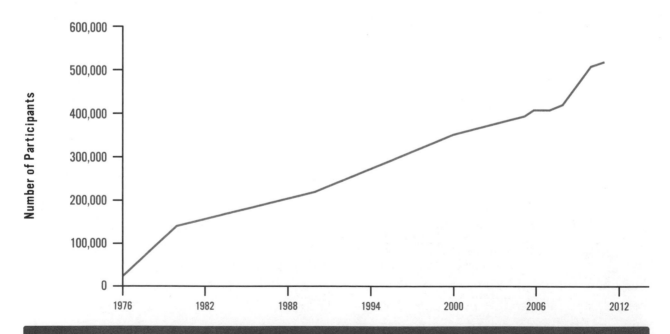

THE MARATHON TREND
Figure 3.1: Popularity of marathon running in the United States from 1975 to 2011. [90]

had Bassler's nod of approval to eat whatever you wanted. Anyone who trained to the point of being able to finish a marathon, he said, was permanently immune to heart attack.[88]

High on promises of invincibility, running enthusiasts embraced Bassler's widely publicized claim, including Jim Fixx, who in the same year (1977) wrote the bestseller *The Complete Book of Running*.[89]

Advocates of aerobics painted a pretty picture: Do a moderate amount of running, swimming, or cycling every week and you're in good shape; do a high amount and you're practically invincible.

But here's the harsh truth that eventually ended Fixx's life: Endurance athletes aren't immune to cardiac incidents. When marathon medical directors reported the number of cardiac events during U.S. marathons from 1976 to 2009, some interesting findings emerged.[91] Across more than 1.5 million participants, there were seven cardiac-related fatalities and roughly two dozen nonfatal cardiac arrests. Although cardiac arrest rates are much higher in the general population, it is worth noting that most of these runners fell victim in the last few miles of the race. Most sudden cardiac arrests happened after mile marker fifteen. More than half occurred within four miles

(6.4 km) of the finish line, calling into question whether they would have occurred under circumstances of less extreme exertion.

Across all cases of fatal and nonfatal cardiac arrest, 93 percent of victims were male, and the mean age was fifty years old.

It brings us to an important question: Why are men twenty times more likely than women to die while exercising?[92] After all, both men and women are susceptible to heart disease. In fact, since 1984, more women than men die of cardiovascular diseases each year.[93] But people tend to think guys' tickers are at higher risk, and that might be because men are affected at a younger age: Heart disease is more likely to strike in middle age for males than females. And this, in turn, might be why rates of sudden cardiac death during exercise are so much higher for men.

It could also be related to other reasons men die earlier in general. Women live about five years longer, on average, notes Dr. Robert H. Shmerling.[94] Statistics show that men often take bigger risks, which could include overdoing it physically. Men are less likely to visit the doctor than women, too, which could mean exacerbating an undiagnosed heart condition through strenuous exercise.

Experienced endurance athletes, such as Brian Maxwell, Jim Fixx, and Micah True, might have ignored early warning signs of trouble and rejected cautionary advice from doctors.[95-96] Perhaps they neglected to schedule medical check-ups at all, despite a family

HEART DISEASE 101

Globally, more people die from cardiovascular diseases (CVD) than from any other cause. CVDs are the number one cause of death in America and the number one cause of premature death. There are two types of cardiovascular disease: **coronary** (ischemic) and **cerebrovascular**. When studies talk about "heart disease," they usually refer to the former, which is also considered the more preventable with lifestyle behaviors, including exercise.

People sometimes mistakenly believe they're immune to cardiovascular complications because they run marathons—but there are many CVD risk factors we can't outrun, including tobacco use, poor diet, obesity, excessive alcohol consumption, genetic predisposition, and previously existing conditions.[100]

A common claim about endurance exercise is that it lessens the risk of coronary heart disease by preventing damage to the coronary arteries. Damage includes **arteriosclerosis**, thickening and hardening of the arteries, and **atherosclerosis**, a type of arteriosclerosis with fat and cholesterol buildup (plaque) along artery walls.[101] Hardening plaque narrows the coronary arteries, which reduces oxygen-rich blood flow to the heart; aerobic exercise, some believe, widens the arteries and preserves their elasticity.

While **anaerobic activity** requires short bursts of higher exertion and we run out of breath quickly (think HIIT and strength training), **aerobic activity** requires consuming a lot of oxygen over a continuous period (i.e., steady-state cardio). Potentially, sustained aerobic exercise brings more oxygen into the blood and widens the arteries, delivering more oxygen-rich blood back to the heart and lungs. Some, such as Dr. Cooper, postulated this trains the heart and lungs to work more efficiently, reducing the heart's "workload," or stress.[102]

Whether this necessarily affects heart health or helps prevent coronary heart disease, however, is not fully known. Many experts suggest the protective benefits could come from other effects of exercise, such as favorable impacts on body fat, diabetes and prediabetes, high blood cholesterol and triglyceride levels, and psychological stress.[103]

history of heart disease and, in the case of Fixx, a prior smoking habit on top of it.[97]

Many symptoms of cardiovascular complications are silent, making themselves first known at heart attack, or worse, sudden death. To put all your money on exercise for heart health is dangerous for anyone, but it becomes even riskier after age thirty-five or for someone with poor lifestyle habits. The same goes for anyone with a family history of heart, lung, or other chronic conditions.[98]

Perhaps taking medical precautions could have saved the lives of Jim Fixx and the other legendary runners whose time was cut too short. You can't outrun a bad diet or any other major risk factor for heart disease. You might be able to buy some extra years of life back. Then again, you might not. Yet, claims about extreme endurance activity and "invincibility" still persist.

While covering the International Marathon in Baghdad in 2016, a *New York Times* correspondent observed a runner poised at the starting line, smoking a cigarette. Running "keeps my health in good standing," the marathoner explained.[99] I don't think anyone ever explicitly said that a person could outrun the deleterious effects of smoking (even Dr. Bassler stopped short of that). But plenty of people think so. Many more believe they can use cardio to reverse a bad diet. We all have the friend who regularly vows to double his laps at the pool tomorrow to "work off" a pizza and beer binge. Maybe it's you.

The "cardio confessional" might make you feel good about your unhealthy choices, but the buck stops there.

THE REAL HARBINGERS OF HEART DISEASE

So how do we reconcile the protective effects of exercise shown in the research with the fatal cardiovascular events striking down endurance athletes? First, lowering risk and eliminating it are not the same thing. The fact is, there are many factors that predict cardiovascular risk. Some risk factors appear to be stronger than physical activity; others can't be teased apart from it.[104-106]

Let's look at the Copenhagen City Heart Study. During 1976 to 2000, researchers followed a large random sample of men and women ages twenty to seventy-nine, all healthy at the outset, until death or the end of the study. Their leisure-time physical activity habits were classified into three categories:

1. The "low" group was mostly sedentary and did less than two hours of light activity, such as walking or biking, per week.

2. The "moderate" group did two to four hours of light physical activity.

3. The "high" group did at least four hours of light activity or at least two hours of vigorous activity per week.

Individuals' activity levels stayed fairly constant over the years. In the end, the moderate and high exercisers did, indeed, fare better. Physically active participants had at least 30 percent lower risk of death from coronary heart disease, cancer, and all causes. On average, highly active women lived 6.4 years longer and moderately active women lived 5.5 years longer than sedentary women. Highly active men lived 6.8 years longer and moderately active men lived 4.9 years longer than sedentary men.

It seems we have our answer about exercise and longevity, right? Except that other data from the Copenhagen City Heart Study tell an interesting story: The more active people also exhibited other low-risk factors for coronary heart disease, cancer, and all-cause mortality. For instance, fewer exercisers than non-exercisers had diabetes or high blood pressure. Significantly fewer were overweight. They were less likely to smoke or drink excessively. But what caused what?

Truthfully, research has never shown that regular exercise makes people 100 percent immune to early death from heart complications. Nor has exercise appeared to outpace other major risk factors, such as hypertension and type 2 diabetes, or lifestyle factors such as smoking.[107] And as you'll see in a moment, running data from the Copenhagen study appeared to show diminished longevity benefits from *too* much exercise.

The well-known Framingham Heart Study showed a similar picture of the relationship between exercise and cardiovascular disease.[108] Once again, as activity went up, mortality went down. The effect was only statistically significant in men; however, other population studies have observed protective effects from exercise in women.[109]

After reviewing the Framingham data, Dr. William Kannel and Paul Sorlie concluded that sedentariness appeared less likely to lop off life-years than smoking, obesity, or high blood pressure. Nonetheless, they concluded that there was an obvious protective effect of exercise, both due to its influence on coexisting risk factors and by itself.

In other words, being active is better than being sedentary. Exercise doesn't grant immunity, but it does give us some sort of improvement in heart health.

Which brings us to the next myth.

THE MYTH: AEROBICS IS ALL

As aerobics leaped to popularity, the public was told to think about exercise as having three distinct categories:

- Cardiovascular and pulmonary conditioning
- Balance and flexibility exercise
- Muscle building

"All three have merit," claimed an article in the *Chicago Sun-Times* featuring an interview with Dr. Cooper, "but only cardiovascular and pulmonary conditioning can prolong life, because it is the only kind that can lower your coronary risk factors."

The journalist instructed, "While yoga and weight training are fine, they have to be done in conjunction with, not in place of, a primary aerobic exercise."[110] Americans heard this message for decades, and it remains an influence on exercise behavior and even government guidelines today.

It's wrong. For starters, activities that improve balance and strength are more than "fine" . . . unless you plan to be a permanent fixture in a rocking chair in your golden years. Second, it is not true that only cardiovascular and pulmonary conditioning (i.e., aerobic exercise) can prolong your life. Optimism and psychological well-being are linked with improved cardiovascular health, so *any* exercise can boost your heart health if it alleviates stress and makes you feel happier.[111] In fact, even in the 1960s, researchers believed *joie de vivre* could play a role in the link between physical activity and lower rates of coronary heart disease.[112]

Given that visceral fat is a leading risk factor in heart disease, exercise that helps you reduce excess body fat will also improve your cardiovascular health.[113] And, as we saw in chapter 2, interval exercise and strength training are better at reducing body fat than aerobic exercise.

Finally, studies have shown that both interval exercise and resistance training lower cardiovascular risk, independent of all the reasons I just listed.

Activities that improve balance and strength are more than "fine" . . . unless you plan to be a permanent fixture in a rocking chair in your golden years.

While protection against coronary heart disease is at the core of the claim that exercise adds years to life, it isn't the only factor. Physical activity—aerobic or not—can help you live longer by improving bone health and reducing the risk of diabetes and certain cancers.[114] Muscular strength has been associated with lower all-cause mortality and reduced prevalence of metabolic syndrome.[115]

In patients with coronary artery disease, resistance training aided cardiac rehabilitation by "improving muscular strength, increasing lean body mass, and reducing body fat."[116]

So what about the early studies Dr. Cooper and others used to make the "only aerobics" claim? Did these specifically show that only endurance exercise was associated with less coronary heart disease?

Not exactly. Remember, these studies were largely of occupational physical activity. If we picture what those farmers and other laborers were doing, we probably don't see them swimming, running, or cycling—the supposed three healthiest activities for the heart. More likely, these men were doing something closer to strength training and interval workouts. The influential 1975 longshoremen study specifically credited "repeated bursts of high-energy output" with the "plateau of protection against coronary mortality" that was observed.[117]

And what about the longevity studies that looked at "leisure-time activity"—that is, structured exercise? Were these people running and cycling? Actually, we have no idea. Participants were rarely asked to list what types of activities they did; instead, they simply reported how active they were, in hours and level of exertion. There was no way to know if people were doing "aerobics" or vigorously polishing their Pontiac Firebird every day.

Population studies, such as the Copenhagen City Heart Study, didn't specifically measure cardio. Rather, like many studies, it was any leisure-time physical activity that "causes perspiration or exhaustion." Prompts on the

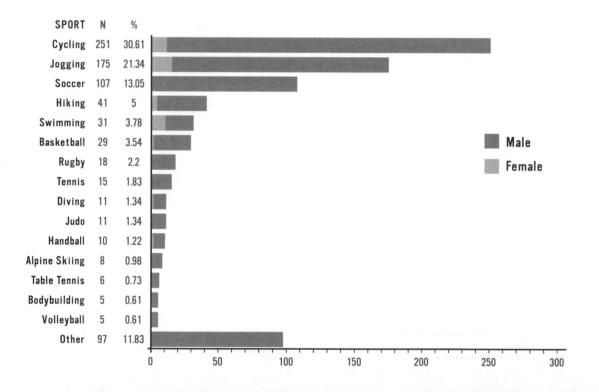

SPORT	N	%
Cycling	251	30.61
Jogging	175	21.34
Soccer	107	13.05
Hiking	41	5
Swimming	31	3.78
Basketball	29	3.54
Rugby	18	2.2
Tennis	15	1.83
Diving	11	1.34
Judo	11	1.34
Handball	10	1.22
Alpine Skiing	8	0.98
Table Tennis	6	0.73
Bodybuilding	5	0.61
Volleyball	5	0.61
Other	97	11.83

Male
Female

SPORTS-RELATED SUDDEN DEATHS IN FRANCE, BY AGE, FROM 2005 TO 2010
Figure 3.2: Most victims of sudden death were middle aged and participating in recreational or "noncompetitive" exercise (more than 90 percent), such as cycling (30.6 percent) and running (21.3 percent); additionally, 95 percent of cases were male.[120]

THE PROBLEM WITH STRESS TESTS

Aerobics was said to condition the heart and lungs to work more efficiently by improving the body's ability to use oxygen. This, according to Dr. Kenneth Cooper, was an indicator that one's cardiovascular system was in good shape. To measure it, Cooper invented the stress test. Essentially, if a patient could run on a treadmill or peddle a stationary bike at max capacity without wobbling, turning pale, running out of breath, or experiencing pain, he passed the stress test, and his heart and lungs were considered healthy.

In addition to testing "fitness," the treadmill test became physicians' primary method for checking the condition of patients' hearts.[121] If one had coronary heart disease, it was supposed to show up in the test, through irregularities in oxygen consumption or the heart's electrical activity, or—with simpler versions of the test—heart rate and blood pressure.

Following this principle, people started administering their own informal stress tests, concluding, "I'm in good shape, because I can run up two flights of stairs without getting winded." But in 1984, cardiologist Henry Solomon took aim squarely at this claim in *The Exercise Myth*. He asserted that passing a fitness test with flying colors didn't mean the absence of heart disease. Nor did it guarantee protection down the road.

"A stress test shows how well you can perform when pushed to work hard during exercise," Solomon explained. "It is a test of function or performance. But coronary heart disease is structural, a narrowing of the coronary arteries that carry oxygen-laden blood to the heart muscle. It is not a disease of performance, and may not interfere with function at all."

Without a doubt, Jim Fixx, Brian Maxwell, and Micah True would all have aced the stress test. Perhaps they had.

questionnaire included brisk walking, fast biking, heavy gardening, and sports.

Which brings up the issue of questionnaires: They aren't considered the epitome of reliability. Even Dr. Cooper admitted this.[118] When reporting typical daily exertion, people might forget to include the ten flights of stairs they always climb to work (less likely) or that their brisk daily walk slows to a crawl when they start daydreaming (more likely).

Basically, it was impossible to say what types of physical activity people in these studies were really doing and if their reported amounts were accurate. Dr. Cooper acknowledged and hoped to fix the issue with his stress test, which would give a foolproof measure of physical fitness. However, critics argued that testing one's cardiorespiratory *fitness* didn't necessarily tell us how much time people spent training, nor everything about their cardiorespiratory *health*.[119]

That physical fitness might be related to lower coronary risk factors (a claim Dr. Cooper made in peer-reviewed publications) did not prove that *aerobics secured heart health* (a claim he made in his books). Guess which claim spread?

Testing one's cardiorespiratory fitness *didn't necessarily tell us how much time people spent training, nor everything about their cardiorespiratory* health.[119]

THE MYTH: MORE IS BETTER

Every day, Dr. Solomon looked out his window and was baffled to see throngs of joggers heading for Central Park. And he couldn't believe there were tens of millions more runners across America doing the same thing. "They seek an unattainable goal," he wrote in *The Exercise Myth*. They have bought into "the mistaken idea that strenuous effort promotes health and longevity."

Despite the "fitness renaissance" and even the rise in marathon running and other extreme endurance sports, the rate of coronary heart disease hadn't declined much since the 1960s.

Dr. Cooper responded: "But if you've got twenty-four million people jogging and it's so dangerous, why aren't we seeing an increased number of deaths from heart attacks? If that had happened, I would have written *The Exercise Myth* myself."

Indeed, as Cooper pointed out, the streets weren't full of dead joggers. Though they weren't *free* of them, either. Looking for trends in the dosage of physical activity, researchers noticed a pattern: Exercise benefits incrementally increased up to a point and then dropped off.

"The findings suggest a U-shaped association between all-cause mortality and dose of jogging," suggested Dr. Peter Schnohr and his colleagues, after homing in on running data from the Copenhagen City Heart Study.[122] Jogging "dose" is calibrated by pace, quantity, and frequency of jogging. "Light and moderate joggers have lower mortality than sedentary nonjoggers," they concluded, "whereas strenuous joggers have a mortality rate not statistically different from that of the sedentary group."

Not only did high doses of cardio not appear to be better, research now suggested it might be as dangerous as doing nothing at all.

Call it the "exercise paradox." Several studies found that exercise occasionally *increased* the risk of keeling over,[123-125] which caused many to ask: Did Jim Fixx, Micah True, and Brian Maxwell exercise themselves to death? There is probably no way to tell. But what we do know is that high-volume running wasn't life insurance.

That said, sudden cardiac death occurs more often in those who exercise infrequently.[126] Sudden cardiac death is less common among competitive runners than recreational ones. The annual death rate is estimated to be somewhere around one to two deaths per 100,000 marathoners, whereas it is thirteen in 100,000 for leisure-time joggers.

In other words, if you're exercising for heart health, you are better off going for a light jog a few times a week than going all out on the treadmill to catch up after a weeklong couch-a-thon.

While *regular* exercise is better, that doesn't mean *excessive* exercise is better. It gets riskier with age, according to cardiologists James O'Keefe, Peter Schnohr, and Carl Lavie.[127] In an editorial in the journal *Heart*, they cautioned individuals against chronic exercise doses, especially after age forty-five or fifty, as "the potential for CV [cardiovascular] damage secondary to extreme endurance exercise appears to increase." They also cautioned against participating in marathons and other extreme endurance events when the aim is health benefits.

While regular *exercise is better, that doesn't mean* excessive *exercise is better.*

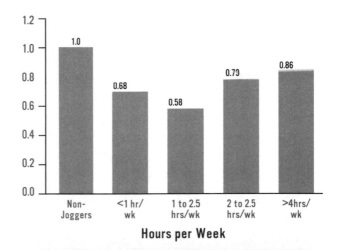

Figure 3.3: Mortality rates in the Copenhagen City Heart Study, with respect to *hours spent* jogging.[128] The risk reduction benefit of running follows a U-shaped curve with 1 being the reference point of non-joggers. See the original study for confidence intervals.

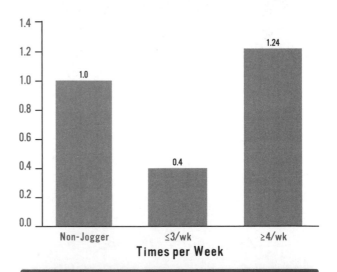

Figure 3.4: Mortality rates in the Copenhagen City Heart Study, with respect to *frequency* of jogging.[129] The risk reduction benefit of running follows a U-shaped curve.

THE GOOD NEWS

By this point, you might be wondering: Why exercise at all?

Here's why. Because the research shows that people who exercise regularly *are* living longer, enjoying life more, and suffering from fewer chronic diseases. It's simply not a cure all, and the benefits aren't limited to aerobics.

It would be ridiculous to claim that only endurance cardio provides stress-reducing benefits, leads to an improved sense of well-being, or motivates people to quit smoking and eat healthier (although that didn't stop some aerobics fanatics from making that claim). Just look at Jack LaLanne, who did strength workouts every day, right up until his ninety-sixth birthday.

At the end of the day, the only exercise that *won't* deliver disease prevention benefits is one you can't stick with. As you'll see in coming chapters, high volumes of endurance exercise pose certain drawbacks, and even health risks, that could negate any longevity reward.

And, if you think you can outrun a daily helping of french fries, six-pack of beer, or pack of cigarettes, go directly to chapter 9 now.

At the end of the day, the only exercise that won't deliver disease prevention benefits is one you can't stick with.

WOMEN, EXERCISE, AND HEART HEALTH

Time to bust another myth! Heart disease is not a "man's disease." In the United States, cardiovascular disease (CVD) remains the leading cause of death for women, as well as men. Although the prevalence of *coronary* heart disease is greater in men, women bear the greater burden of overall *cardiovascular* disease, which encompasses coronary heart disease, heart failure, and strokes.[83]

Premature CVD is relatively rare in women under fifty-five, the American Heart Association reports. One reason for the older onset in females might be a decrease in estrogen levels after menopause. Estrogen is believed to offer a protective effect up to that point. Still, more women than men die from heart disease each year—a fact that the American Heart Association strives to raise awareness about.[84]

The good news is that women can reap protective benefits from exercise, just like the guys. Population studies like the Nurses' Health Study, established in 1976, observed that physical activity was associated with reduced risk of coronary heart disease. When coupled with a healthy diet and not smoking, the risk was very low.[85]

PART

2

WHAT YOU NEED TO KNOW

- When people talk about the longevity benefits of exercise, they are primarily talking about lowering the risk of coronary heart disease. Whether this occurs from increased efficiency of the heart and lungs or from other factors is not fully known.

- Systematic reviews of the evidence repeatedly show that people who exercise regularly tend to live longer than sedentary people. However, the data rarely includes measures of the types of exercise people are doing. There are also confounding factors: Exercisers tend to exhibit other healthy behaviors.

- There appears to be a point of diminishing returns with cardio exercise, after which, studies suggest, it becomes less beneficial for the heart and, even, potentially dangerous. After age forty or fifty, individuals are cautioned against extreme exercise.

THE
MINOR
MYTHS

120 minutes of HIIT delivers an aerobic endurance boost equivalent to 1,800 minutes of cycling.

4

GOING THROUGH THE MOTIONS:
WHY CARDIO FAILS THE HUMAN NATURE TEST

IT NEVER CEASES to amaze me what people will come up with to occupy their minds while doing cardio exercise they don't enjoy. Some read books; others try to read the newspaper while seated on a recumbent bike, awkwardly struggling to turn the pages while pedaling. Others, thanks to the advent of smart phones, check their email, hold business conference calls, surf the web, watch movies, or play games. Today, you can even find equipment that has the Internet built into the screen.

One woman at a gym where I was a trainer sticks out in my mind. She must have gone through three Hollywood gossip magazines during each cardio session. Her exercise pace was abysmal. She couldn't have walked slower up an icy hill. There's no way her thirty-minute workout could have burned a hundred calories. I can't imagine what she expected from such little effort, or perhaps she was so engrossed in her reading that she actually thought she was exercising at a decent pace. Five days a week; a year later, there's no change.

She's not the only one. There are millions like her, men and women alike, who struggle with their pooches and potbellies, never getting anywhere, and doing nothing more than wasting time and making dirty clothes for the laundry bin.

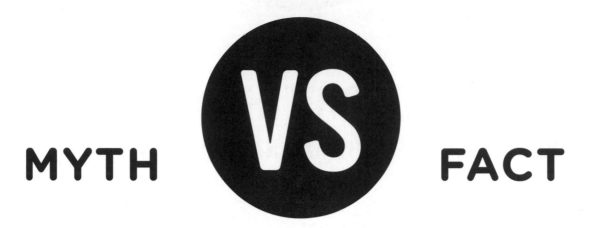

MYTH VS FACT

MYTH	FACT
Exercising at a low or moderate intensity, at a continuous pace, will deliver the best fat loss and aerobic endurance benefits.	Varying your intensity is often a more effective way to get results. Think peaks and valleys, if you were looking at a cardio machine monitor, rather than a steady level of intensity.
There's nothing wrong with watching TV or reading while getting your daily exercise in.	Multitasking can foster low exertion and poor form. Low focus and low exertion are two reasons cardio, especially when done on a machine, fails to deliver benefits.
A person needs to exercise for at least twenty minutes before fat burning kicks in.	The fat-burning zone idea is misleading, and studies have proven that people can lose fat with as little as four minutes of high-intensity exercise per week!
When it comes to exercise and results, more is better.	When it comes to exercise for fat loss, *better* is better! Quality matters more for results than quantity.

If the appeal of a workout is that it's so easy you can do other things at the same time . . . beware. Sure, it's killing two birds with one stone. But those birds are your *fitness results* and *precious time*. This chapter reveals why human nature—in the form of physiological and behavioral quirks—has so many cardio exercisers spinning their wheels.

If the appeal of a workout is that it's so easy you can do other things at the same time . . . beware.

THE HUMAN NATURE TEST

When it comes to exercise, there are two facts about humans that we just can't run from.

We are, by nature, a bit lazy. (If that seems harsh, bear with me—as you're about to discover, we're *hardwired* to conserve energy, so it's not totally our fault.) There's something I call the human nature test. I made it up, but it goes like this: If you give people the choice between two tasks, nine times out of ten, they will choose the easier one. For example, if you put one hundred people in a gym, ninety will flock to the cardio machines. Of those, 90 percent will pick the elliptical machine because it is the easiest. That's why cardio machines outnumber resistance-training equipment by ten or twenty to one in most fitness centers.

Which brings me to the second fact about humans: We are not very good at multitasking. Cardio makes it easy to do two things at once. It's so brain-dead simple: just put one foot in front of the other and go. It requires little thought or exertion to keep moving, which makes it easy to direct focus elsewhere—and most people do.

I know several people who use their morning jog or elliptical session as their thinking time, when they meditate on life goals or work through the day's problems. Others find the monotony excruciatingly dull and take advantage of the opportunity to multitask (or pretend they're not exercising) by reaching for their phone, book, or TV remote.

But you know what they say: Chase two rabbits, catch none. Neuroscientists have been telling us for years that humans are not good at multitasking.[130] Our noggins simply aren't built for it, even though we think they are, and tech-gadget marketers spend billions of dollars a year reinforcing that belief.[131]

You may start out at a steady clip, but as soon as that e-book gets good, your pace is going to slow to a crawl. But there's another problem with zoning out.

Consider this: Talking on the phone with a handheld device while driving is currently outlawed in fourteen states.[132] Why? Because it quadruples the likelihood of a car accident.[133] Some studies have even found that the effect of using technology while operating a car is similar to driving drunk.[134]

CALORIES 101

Calorie: This is a unit used to measure energy, for example, potential energy from food. If you consume more energy than your body uses, it gets stored in the body and you gain weight. So, when a machine or monitor tells you how many calories you're burning, this is a proxy for how much energy it thinks you're using.

Metabolism: This is, essentially, how many calories your body burns each day. You'll also hear the term *energy expenditure*, which basically describes the same thing. Your daily calorie burn comes from three processes.

- **Basal metabolic rate** or **resting metabolic rate**, which accounts for roughly 70 percent of a person's daily calorie expenditure, and refers to the number of calories the body uses at rest for basic functions, such as blood circulation and growing and repairing cells[136]

- **Thermogenesis**, which is the digesting, transporting, and storing the food you eat.

- **Physical activity:** The number of calories the body needs for physical activity varies the most, while calories used for thermogenesis and resting metabolism are fairly constant but influenced by certain factors, such as genetics and body size and composition.

    Across the board, muscle mass is the biggest contributor to metabolic rate.[137] Muscle tissue burns more calories than fat tissue, which is why losing muscle mass slows metabolism, and, conversely, increasing muscle can speed it up.

Machine calorie counters, such as those on an exercise machine, don't actually tell you how many calories you're burning; rather, it's an *estimate* based on predicted energy expenditure given the following equation:

$$\text{amount of time} \times \text{a given intensity}$$

Now, the bad news: Those estimates are fraught with error. Methods for measuring energy expenditure in a lab are much more complex, and some machines are notoriously bad at giving accurate readings (more in chapter 6).

It's the same with multitasking during exercise. Beyond low exertion, the distractedness that ensues during continuous-paced exertion—whether caused by technology or being lulled into a daydream—means attention is no longer paid to maintaining proper form or observing your surroundings. Running seems to lend itself to more injuries than other types of leisure exercise; even when you limit yourself to the treadmill, chances are still high you might hurt yourself.[135] Walking is probably safer than running simply because if you're going to twist an ankle or trip on a jagged sidewalk edge, the wreckage will be lesser at a lower speed.

But we'll save the gory details of cardio-related injuries for chapter 5. For now, let's turn to the physiological reasons that putting in your cardio time rarely produces the lean, strong, toned figure people are expecting.

CALORIES IN, CALORIES OUT? IF ONLY!

Wait a minute. A calorie burned is a calorie burned, right? Say you commit to exercising for a certain amount of time and stay focused. The machine says you're burning 200 calories. Then shouldn't you expect to get the same results—no matter what type of exercise you're doing, at what speed, or how long it takes?

Nice try. If only it were that simple. But few things ever are when it comes to the human body, and exercise is no exception. The relationship between physical activity and fat loss has proven—time and again—to be more complicated than a simple calorie balance equation.

Here's the thing. *Amount* of exercise and *intensity* of exercise are not created equal. Though you might expend the same amount of energy in a long, slow workout as an intense, short one, each will produce a different metabolic response in the body. Herein lies the crux of why your level of exertion matters for fat loss.

Amount *of exercise and* intensity *of exercise are not created equal.*

RESEARCH RECAP: CARDIO VERSUS HIIT FOR FAT LOSS

Remember the (rather depressing) study from chapter 2, in which six hours of moderate to vigorous cardio a week produced a fat loss of only four to six pounds (1.8 to 2.7 kg) in an entire year?[138] Well, a meta-analysis of steady-state cardio studies found the same thing. Across twenty-eight studies, men lost an average of 6.6 pounds (3 kg) from thirty weeks of aerobic exercise. Women shed, on average, a paltry 3 pounds (1.4) in thirteen weeks.[139] Further, the cardio failed to affect their fat-free mass, meaning it didn't help them increase muscle.

> *Those who regularly did intense activity had a more favorable waist-to-hip ratio and lower subcutaneous skinfold thickness, despite spending much less time exercising.*

Meanwhile, studies that compared HIIT to cardio found that the high-intensity interval exercisers were losing more fat. When Dr. Tremblay and his colleagues analyzed large amounts of data from the Canada Fitness Survey, they found that people engaging in higher-intensity activity had better body composition than endurance exercisers, overall.[140] Those who regularly did intense activity had a more favorable waist-to-hip ratio and lower subcutaneous skinfold thickness (meaning they could pinch less fat), despite spending much less time exercising.

Now, this information was gathered by a survey, which is never completely reliable. But numerous controlled lab experiments have led to the same conclusion.[141-143] Short HIIT workouts consistently do better at significantly reducing total body fat and unhealthy visceral fat.[144] Even two sessions a week of HIIT plus one resistance training session have led to documented significant improvements in body fat percentage, visceral fat mass, and reduction in waist size.[145]

In most HIIT studies, researchers control for energy expenditure. That means they analyze the effects of cardio and HIIT regimens given equal energy expenditure. Even with matching energy output in Dr. Tremblay's famous 1994 study, subjects in the HIIT group had nine times the subcutaneous fat loss as the cardio group. Similarly, as Dr. Tremblay noted, high-intensity interval exercise has led to greater fat loss than cardio in some studies despite *lower* energy expenditure.

Before we solve the mystery of why more exercise doesn't automatically lead to more fat burn, let's detour to a related and equally pressing question: What kept our ancestors fit?

THE EVOLUTIONARY ARGUMENT

There are two main camps in the debate over exercise evolution. One says that humans evolved to do long bouts of low-exertion activity, roving the plains to gather food all day. The other view is that humans evolved to function optimally with short bursts of intense movement, spending much of their time conserving energy, until it was time to hunt for food or run for their lives from a predator.

Which is correct? Well, it's entirely possible that *both* patterns of daily exertion kept our ancestors in top shape. However, it doesn't really matter because all this was before the advent of the Western lifestyle.

We live in a different world today, and it's simply not enough to imitate what our predecessors might have done for exercise.

We're fending off new threats, such as highly processed and calorie-packed foods, jumbo portion sizes, pizza crusts stuffed with cheese and hot dogs, sedentary jobs, cars and elevators, and chronic stressors. It all affects our waistlines—as does the nearby chair that's always available to sit down in. In other words, we have to adapt.

Let's pause to consider that, over the last three decades, exercise rates and obesity rates have risen in tandem. Despite the popularity of cardio activities such as walking, jogging, bicycling, and aerobics, body mass indexes (BMIs) are still on the rise.

You might say it's because we're eating more calories, and that's definitely true. But surely exercise could help stave off the weight gain . . . if exercise worked the way people think it does.

It seems obvious that while our ancestors may have done a whole lot of walking—or that we may have even been "born to run" (which I doubt, but we'll get to that in chapter 5)—the whole sixty to ninety minutes of moderate daily cardio isn't going to keep us slim in the twenty-first century. But you don't have to take my word for it—take Dr. Herman Pontzer's. He is the anthropologist behind a series of studies that say, essentially, just that.

The latest study to come out of Pontzer's lab has gotten plenty of media buzz, and it's no wonder. It revealed that—beyond a certain threshold—energy output from exercise simply plateaus.[146] At least that's how it appeared in data from a large, mixed-sex sample of people drawn from five populations in Africa and North America. After comparing their daily amounts of physical activity and energy

MEAN	HAZDA WOMEN	HAZDA MEN	WESTERN WOMEN	WESTERN MEN
Weight	95.7	112.2	164	178.6
BMI	20.2	20.3	27.5	25.6
Body Fat Percent	20.9	13.5	37.9	22.5
Energy Expenditure (kCal/day)	1,877	2,649	2,347	3,053

ENERGY EXPENDITURE IN WESTERN AND HAZDA GROUPS
Figure 4.1: Despite walking up to twice as far per day, the Tanzanian foragers—the Hazda—in Dr. Pontzer's study burned fewer daily calories than the Westerners.

expenditure, the scientists found these only corresponded *up to a point*.

Past that threshold, activity continued to rise ... energy expenditure did not.

That sounds strange, right? Why wouldn't more exercise lead to more calories burned? And here's where the plot thickens.

Beyond a certain threshold—energy output from exercise simply plateaus.[146]

Humans appear to have a built-in system for conserving energy. In another study, Pontzer compared the daily physical activity of Westerners and the Hazda, an indigenous tribe of hunter-gatherers in north-central Tanzania whose present-day lifestyle mirrors our foraging ancestors.[147] The Hazda had higher physical activity levels than your typical Westerner. However, energy expenditure was about the same in both groups.

"We found that despite all this physical activity, the number of calories the Hazda burned per day was indistinguishable from that of typical adults in Europe and the United States," Pontzer explained.[148]

It's kind of neat, actually. This mechanism could prevent you from wasting away, should you have to forage far and wide for food during a famine. But it could also prevent you from walking off tons of extra pounds.

Suddenly, all those studies showing minimal weight loss from cardio are starting to make sense, aren't they? The body adapts to prevent extreme energy expenditure, which is why doing ninety minutes a day of cardio won't help you get better results than doing forty-five minutes ... and forty-five minutes, as we've seen, won't get you much fat loss to begin with.

DOES THAT MEAN ALL EXERCISE IS POINTLESS?

Don't give up on your fitness goals and take a torch to your exercise gear just yet. The news headlines proclaiming that exercise has been proven unnecessary, even "futile," are merely meant to grab your attention. I can only hope people read the actual articles, wherein every reporter backpedals from the shock-headline claim and concludes that exercise is still important.[149] The research still says so.[150] Even Dr. Pontzer thinks so.

No, exercise is not pointless. Well, not *all* exercise. When large, systematic reviews of the evidence have led to the "don't bother" conclusion, they've usually drawn almost exclusively on studies of cardio exercise.[151] As for the Hazda people, their top activity is walking.

But a quick glance back at the myriad HIIT studies should revive your optimism. Obviously, people *can* and *do* lose fat with exercise. So how do we get around the energy expenditure plateau?

Part of the secret is controlling the behavioral mechanisms that offset results. Researchers have identified several such sneaky habits (often connected specifically to cardio) and there's a whole chapter coming up on that.

So, for now, let's look at how to avoid the plateau effect *physiologically*. What do Pontzer's findings tell us? That lots of moderate steady-state cardio—the standard form of physical activity—won't lead to expending lots of energy. Instead, fat loss depends on exercise that can help you simultaneously expend energy, build muscle, and increase your resting metabolic rate, or how many calories you burn when you're not exercising.

Three components of an exercise regimen dictate whether you'll achieve these results: intensity, variety, and change. A regimen based on these criteria is more likely to produce different and better metabolic changes in the body, leading to superior fat loss.

Let's start with the most important factor—the intensity of your exercise.

WHY INTENSITY MATTERS FOR FAT LOSS

For every person who is oblivious to their low-intensity workout because they're distracted, another is intentionally taking it easy because they read somewhere that slow and steady wins the race. It doesn't. Especially not for fat loss.

Some people have been misguided by the fat-burning zone myth (see sidebar, page 75

for more on that). And, from time to time, you'll hear the media or some health organization claim that walking is a great fat burner. Perhaps they've been looking at studies, such as the one from Wake Forest University School of Medicine, in which the pounds dropped significantly in a group of treadmill walkers who were obese[152]—keyword, *obese*.

As you've learned in previous chapters, the more weight you have to lose, the easier it comes off when you start exercising . . . at first. Part of the reason is that when you're overweight, you're bearing more weight, so the energy cost of walking is higher. But after losing some of that weight, your body expends less energy to do the same activity.[153] Hence, the disheartening recommendation that formerly obese individuals would need to increase their physical activity to "eighty to ninety minutes of moderate levels of activity, such as walking or cycling" per day to maintain their results.[154]

What should all this data tell us? That walking is not an effective long-term strategy for fat loss or preventing fat gain. It definitely doesn't tell us that people should double or triple their walking time to get the results they got in the beginning—or the results reported in studies of only obese walkers.

We know that studies of the effects of low- to moderate-intensity exercise in non-obese people continually show meager fat loss results. A systematic review of the research published in the esteemed Cochrane Library concluded that *increased intensity* leads to *increased weight loss*.[155] Sticking with a low-intensity routine is a common reason for weight regain. After a certain point in your fat loss journey, you're going to need to kick it up a notch. It's plain and simple.

It's here that some people will loop back around to the argument that intense exertion uses more energy in a given timeframe, which could mean that high-intensity *cardio* is just as good as high-intensity *intervals* for fat loss. Is it? I'm glad you asked.

Some studies have, indeed, found that running works better than walking to reduce abdominal fat in, say, obese middle-aged women.[156] However, other studies have found zero weight loss difference between moderate- and high-intensity cardio, given equal duration.[157-158]

Sticking with a low-intensity routine is a common reason for weight regain. After a certain point in your fat loss journey, you're going to need to kick it up a notch. It's plain and simple.

The reason for the lack of difference could come down to a flawed way of classifying "intensity." Participants in one of these studies were classified as having either moderate- or high-intensity activities, such as badminton, but how intense does your backyard badminton really get?

Here's another example of classification blurriness. One study compared intense aerobic dance to walking and found that the high-intensity group came out fitter.[159] But a closer look reveals that they weren't really doing steady-state cardio at all. It was a combination of aerobic dance and stepping with a step bench.

In this study, subjects performed the aerobic dance at a level that raised their heart rate from 70 to 85 percent of their maximum (they rated their exertion level from "fairly hard" to "very hard"), and the steps progressed to advanced lunges by the end of the session. That looks like a HIIT workout, not an aerobic workout, if you ask me!

We can also note that, although both groups lost some weight at the end of fourteen weeks, only the group that was doing the "aerobic dance workout" (which was actually a high-intensity interval workout plus a bodyweight component) managed to preserve lean body mass.

The walkers, on the other hand, lost muscle.

In Pontzer's most recent study, exercise categories were based on total amount of energy expended. Although the researchers categorized physical activity levels as either "vigorous" or "sedentary," *intensity* of activity was not measured—only duration. Thus it is possible—and actually, highly probable—that most people in the "vigorous" category were simply doing a lot of low- to moderate-intensity activity.

THE MYTH OF THE FAT-BURNING ZONE

Some people think they need to pass the twenty-minute mark in a workout before they even start burning fat. Guess that rules out four-minute HIIT workouts for fat loss, right?

Hardly. In reality, you're always burning fat, even while you sit on the couch, and especially when you do a short burst workout.

The other half of the fat-burning zone myth has to do with intensity. Specifically, the idea is that optimal fat burn occurs at around 60 percent of your maximum exertion, which is based on your oxygen consumption. According to the theory, going at 60 percent of your capacity is somehow better than 80 percent. Now, it may be the case that during lower exertion (e.g., jogging leisurely) a greater *proportion* of the calories you burn comes from fat than protein or carbohydrates, compared to higher exertion. But that's misleading. The fact is, you still burn more calories total—and more calories from fat—during a high-intensity workout than a low-intensity one of the same duration. Here's a table to demonstrate.

TOTAL CALORIES BURNED TRUMPS PERCENT OF CALORIES FROM FAT
Figure 4.2: Source: www.pinoyfitness.com/?p=8

ACTIVITY	CALORIES BURNED	FAT PERCENTAGE	CALORIES FROM FAT
Watching TV for 30 Minutes	50	70%	35
Jogging for 30 Minutes	150	60%	90
Sprinting for 30 Minutes	300	40%	120

Don't let this myth fool you into thinking that a forty-five-minute saunter through the park will deliver any fat-burning zone advantage compared with a ten-minute high-intensity interval workout. The research has proven this false.

DID YOU KNOW HIIT CAN BOOST AEROBIC ENDURANCE?

Unless you're training for an endurance sport, you don't really need aerobic training. As explained in chapter 3, aerobic capacity is not necessarily an indicator of heart health. But let's say you want to improve your aerobic endurance—you're training for a charity relay race and don't want to embarrass the team. Good news: You still don't have to chain yourself to a treadmill for sixty minutes a day!

In the Tokyo lab of Dr. Izumi Tabata, back in the mid-1990s, two groups of men exercised on stationary bikes for five workouts a week for six weeks.[161] One group did a sixty-minute cycling workout. The other did an explosive HIIT workout, pedaling at maximum effort for twenty seconds, followed by ten seconds of rest. The cycle was repeated for a total of four minutes.

After six weeks, the four-minute HIIT program produced a level of aerobic conditioning comparable to the endurance-training program. The regular cardio group logged 1,800 minutes of cycling, while the HIIT group logged just 120 minutes. The HIIT protocol led to the same boost in aerobic capacity—in just 7 percent of the time.

This breakthrough marked the birth of the four-minute workout concept. Not only did Tabata's HIIT exercisers have an increase in *aerobic* capacity, they also upped their *anaerobic* capacity, while the endurance group did not. Tabata's team concluded that high-intensity intervals tax both the aerobic and anaerobic systems maximally. In other words, a six-week HIIT regimen could prepare you for both a relay run and sprinting to the beer tent when it's over.

As Pontzer had concluded after his earlier study of the Hazda people (see page 71), the "hunter-gatherer workout"—which primarily consists of a great deal of walking—is not your best bet for weight loss.[160] High-intensity cardio, such as running or cycling at a fast pace, is indeed probably better for fat loss than walking. But it might not be worth the cost. It would be difficult to maintain your full-throttle pace for very long and doing so might result in injury, as you'll see in chapter 5. Recall from chapter 3 that longevity benefits also diminish in exercisers who regularly run or cycle at a strenuous pace.

Besides, although many would surely argue that running marathons is "intense," long strenuous bouts of exercise do not appear to have the same fat loss benefits as HIIT. In chapter 6, I'll show you why it's not uncommon for people to gain weight—much to their surprise—while training for a marathon.

That brings us to the advantage of intervals.

THE MAGIC OF INTERVALS

High-intensity interval training is consistently superior for fat loss in the research, which points to physiological responses that are unique to the interval nature of HIIT: alternating between short bursts of very intense activity and periods of rest.[162]

A huge predictor in whether your workout will help you lose fat is what happens *after* the workout. A thirty-minute elliptical session might burn 200 calories during the workout (if you trust the counter), but it won't do much to raise your metabolism afterward, which is where the bigger, long-term fat loss results come from. And metabolism, in turn, is influenced by how your exercise regimen affects your muscle mass.

We saw in chapter 2 that steady-state cardio does little to preserve muscle mass and sometimes even depletes it. HIIT, on the other hand, has been found to either preserve muscle or build it—and that's true whether you're doing an HIIT strength-training circuit or high-intensity interval cardio, such as sprints on a stationary bike.

It's not enough to alternate between medium and low intensity. Nor do the beneficial effects of HIIT apply to other types of "intermittent exercise," such as splitting a longer cardio workout into two shorter ones. In one study, subjects who split their thirty-minute walk into two fifteen-minute walks a day, not surprisingly, still got dismal fat loss results.[163]

The key, again, is the combination of high intensity and intervals. The reasons that HIIT increases post-exercise energy consumption aren't fully understood.[164] But the research suggests this: By alternating short bursts of intense activity with rest, you're severely stressing the metabolic capabilities of your muscle cells and, thus, burning more fat for energy.

There are several things happening that could contribute to greater fat loss and energy consumption:

1. HIIT burns a lot of muscle glycogen (stored carbohydrates), and the body burns energy to refill those stores.

2. HIIT increases growth hormone levels, and growth hormone is a natural fat-burning hormone.

3. Intervals increase protein turnover in muscle cells—that is, the healthy breakdown and rebuilding of muscle tissue—which is an energy-intensive process that causes a lot of calorie burning after exercise.

Think of it like running a factory at full tilt, making the conveyor belts go faster and faster. Intervals exhaust the energy stores of the muscle fiber faster, just as you'd exhaust the supplies of the factory by turning up the conveyor belt. And when you finally slow down, during your recovery from short burst exercise bouts, the factory workers have to work hard to stock up supplies again. This constant accelerated work rate leads to more work being done, and, in the body, that means more calories burned during the hard exercise bout and then during the recovery.

High-intensity interval training is so efficient that men have even lost fat in four minutes of full-intensity sprinting per week.[165]

This post-workout recovery calorie burning is colloquially known as "afterburn," and the entire concept was the basis for Turbulence Training, the program I developed (and named while riding through turbulence on a flight from Salt Lake City to Toronto in 2001). Essentially, you are putting "turbulence" on the body during the exercise session, and, when you recover, your body is in afterburn mode for hours (and some claim days), burning more calories and causing greater fat loss.

High-intensity interval training is so efficient that men have even lost fat in four minutes of full-intensity sprinting *per week*.[165] Not including the short warm-ups and rest periods, that's a total of eighty seconds of intense exercise per workout. Three times a week. For a grand total of just four minutes.

There's yet another reason that varying your workout pace is important. As Dr. Pontzer's studies revealed, we're hardwired as humans to try to conserve energy. A workout that demands focus will help you prevent an unconscious workout lull.

HOW TO RATE INTENSITY

"Intensity" refers to how physical exertion affects *your* body. Your "moderate" and "vigorous" might be different from someone else's! Here's a simple way to think about it:

Low intensity = *little to no* change in your breathing or heart rate

Moderate intensity = a *small* change in your breathing or heart rate

Vigorous intensity = a *big* change in your breathing or heart rate

WHY YOU SHOULD CHANGE IT UP

Change is the final secret to success. Periodically changing your workout routine is important for the same reason as varied intensity—it prevents your body from adapting.

Most people do a cardio regimen until it becomes a rut. They repeat their daily walk or run month after month, year after year. It's performed at a continuous low or moderate cadence, without any variation, and the body adapts and stops responding. Either that, or the repetition leads to overuse injuries. I'll explain this more in chapter 8 and give you a great plan for progressing through your exercise regimen.

I recognize that very intense exertion may not be feasible for everyone, such as people with existing medical conditions or injuries who need approval from their doctor. But increasing your intensity is something most individuals can work toward. Intensity level is relative, so "higher" intensity is based on your own capability levels, no one else's.

Let's say you have a lot of excess weight or haven't exercised in years. It's fine to start slower.

As the weight comes off, or you condition your body to move with greater intensity for short bursts, you will increase your capacity for exertion.

Pairing your exercise with a smart nutrition approach, like the one discussed in chapter 9, will help you lose fat.

FOLLOW THE RULE OF THREE IN YOUR WORKOUT

Many people choose cardio because the alternatives, those that actually work, are, quite frankly, harder. Strength training and interval training require you to focus, even though it's only for short bursts. They also require planning and even psyching yourself up to do those push-ups, rather than mindlessly putting one foot in front of the other while gazing at the TVs in the cardio area.

But the results are worth it.

If you want to improve your body composition, choose a workout regimen that incorporates intensity, variety, and change. These principles apply to strength training, too, as you'll see in later chapters.

If you want to improve your body composition, choose a workout regimen that incorporates intensity, variety, and change.

WHAT YOU NEED TO KNOW

- Research consistently suggests that the positive effects of HIIT aren't caused by high intensity alone; rather, it is the combination of short bursts of intensity and rest in an interval format. This could partly be because HIIT does more to preserve muscle mass than endurance cardio (even cardio performed at a high intensity).

- Strength training and interval training require focus, even though only for short bursts, which is another reason they tend to produce better weight loss results.

- Studies show that there is a cap on our daily energy expenditure. After a certain amount of activity, the body finds ways to conserve energy and calorie burn plateaus.

- Exercise that incorporates the rule of three (intensity, variety, and change) seems to circumvent the energy expenditure plateau observed in long cardio workouts.

Up to 92% of runners will eventually get injured while running — usually badly enough to require medical attention.

5

THE FABLED FOUNTAIN OF YOUTH

CATHERINE WAS LIVING her dream. She had quit smoking and given birth to a son, and now she was raising a family with her husband in an idyllic small town in California.

Everything was perfect . . . except physically. Physically, things were going downhill fast. Catherine couldn't lose the extra weight she gained during pregnancy. As you might remember from chapter 1, it wasn't for lack of exercise. For a long time, her dedicated workout regimen included an hour on the treadmill, several days a week. Despite steadily increasing her gym time, she was stuck at 165 pounds (75 kg), which felt heavy on her 5'1" (155 cm) frame.

The extra weight was taking its toll. One day while choreographing a dance number, Catherine demonstrated a big jump and came down hard. Her foot broke in four places. She was distraught. What was she doing wrong? Eventually out of the cast and back on the treadmill again, she worked out harder than ever, but things weren't getting better—they were getting worse.

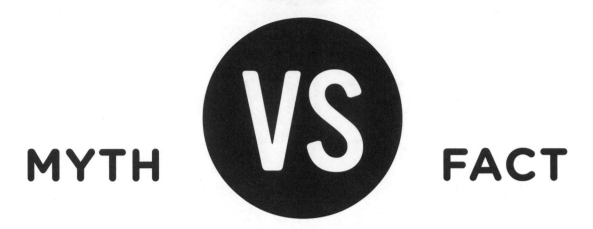

MYTH VS FACT

MYTH	FACT
Running is a primal and natural activity. Humans were born to run.	Humans do not appear to be built for long, repetitive activity. It leads to overuse injuries and wear and tear on the joints, and, in extreme cases, it can overtax the heart.
Cardio is the only exercise that delivers psychological benefits and an endorphin boost.	You can get well-being, stress relief, exercise endorphins, and an energy boost from strength training and interval workouts.
Aerobic activities are the safest kind for middle age and beyond.	High amounts of cardio, especially running, can lead to acute and overuse injuries, which may take longer to heal in older individuals.
The more cardio, the better it is for your health.	Too much cardio can damage the body, increase the production of stress hormones, and have the opposite effect.

The big wake-up call came on a Tuesday around her forty-fourth birthday, when Catherine was shopping at a local grocery store and the cashier asked her a question she'd never forget: "Ma'am, do you qualify for our senior's discount?"

Mistaken for a senior . . . at forty-four? She was mortified.

Ever since the invention of aerobics, cardio has been hailed as revitalizing. Beyond promising slimmer waistlines and healthier hearts, it is sold as a way to improve energy and well-being and keep the body in top condition. So why does it sometimes have a reverse effect?

Obviously, the traditional cardio-based approach to health and fitness wasn't keeping Catherine young. She felt and looked older than ever.

Cardio promised to keep us young, but the science should really have us asking, "Is it a fountain of youth or an age accelerator?"

To a certain extent, it's reasonable to expect that cardio would be a fountain of youth. Exercise, of any kind, is linked with lower risk of disease, more energy, greater productivity, and less stress. But what people haven't been told is that large amounts of cardio can also age us prematurely.

Wait, how can that be? And how did we not know this? It's strange, since scientists have been aware of this paradox for years.

In the scientific literature, very high volumes of cardio have been linked with hormonal disruptions, cardiac damage, brittle bones, and malnutrition. Many endurance athletes—even recreational ones—suffer acute injuries, as well as chronic overuse injuries that get harder to recover from with age.[166]

But somehow the research findings have been swept aside, decade after decade, as long-endurance exercise is continually marketed to the masses as the ideal way to stay in shape. Cardio promised to keep us young, but the science should really have us asking, "Is it a fountain of youth or an age *accelerator*?" There is definitely a cutoff point for benefits— and it may be lower than people think.

THE FIRST GENERATION OF AEROBICS FANS, FIFTY YEARS LATER

While some people exercise in hope of heart health or weight loss, many do it in search of vibrancy, happiness, confidence, and, later in life, independence.

When cardio was introduced to the world, the resounding message was "the more, the better," as Kenneth Cooper explained in his 1968 book *Aerobics*. He reserved top praise for competitive athletes, as well as the recreational exercisers who really pushed themselves.

Cooper maintained that, "The running program, without any equivocation, is the best." Running is fast and easy, he said, and all you need is a pair of running shoes. Running "can be done for the rest of your life," he promised, "and a long, productive life it should be."

Running was supposed to buy a person less illness, better sleep, improved self-image, relaxation, and even work productivity. No wonder people became obsessed with racking up miles, optimistically scooping up more of this life elixir.

Unfortunately, what people got was a mixed bag. Take a comment recently left on the Amazon page for Cooper's original *Aerobics* book (yes, tattered old copies of this outdated guide are still for sale):

> *I started when the book came out in 1968. I initially ran a mile (1.6 km), then worked up to four miles (6.4 km) a day. What the book didn't tell you is that, eventually, it takes a toll on your knees. It may be better now, with well-engineered running shoes to absorb some of the impact, but after about twenty years my knees couldn't take the strain. Arthroscopic surgery, and then a switch to bicycling and a bike machine.*[167]

Not exactly the epitome of youth. Poor guy. And judging by the current research, no, it hasn't gotten any better.

BORN TO RUN OR DIE TRYING?

The odds of sustaining a running injury are high—so high, in fact, it's almost a guarantee.

In a 2007 systematic review of seventeen running injury studies, published in the *British Journal of Sports Medicine*, the incidence of lower-body injuries among runners ranged from 26 percent all the way up to 79.3 percent.[168]

If you include upper-body injuries in the casualty report, the reported incidence in published studies climbed as high as 92.4 percent.

Across all of these studies, the knees took the most beating. Next came the lower legs (shins, Achilles tendons, and calves), the feet, and the upper legs (hamstrings, thighs, and quadriceps). But even ankles, hips, and groins were not spared.

And the following might make you think twice about putting "run a marathon" on your bucket list. At one particular marathon, about 18 percent of runners detoured to the medical aid post with injuries. As for the runners who were off the hook that day, statistics suggest it's only a matter of time.[169]

The two biggest risk factors for sustaining an injury that emerged in the research were long training distances each week and a prior history of injuries. Most runners fill the bill on both counts.

Another recent study echoed the finding that a past injury is a good indicator of a future one.[170] This study, led by Harvard professor Irene Davis, Ph.D., followed 249 experienced

RUNNING INJURIES 101

Runners are prone to certain acute and chronic overuse injuries, especially in the knee (42.1 percent of injured runners) and foot and ankle (16.9 percent).[172] But the damage can be found throughout the lower body, including lower leg (12.8 percent); hip/pelvis (10.9 percent); Achilles/calf (6.4 percent); upper leg (5.2 percent); low back (3.4 percent); and other locations (2.2 percent).

In a case-control analysis of 2,002 running injuries, the ten most common injuries were the following:*

- Patellofemoral pain syndrome (a.k.a. "runner's knee"; pain behind the kneecap); F
- Iliotibial band friction syndrome (pain between the hip and knees); F
- Plantar fasciitis (heel pain); M
- Meniscal injuries (knee cartilage tears); M
- Tibial stress syndrome (shin splints)
- Achilles tendinopathy (pain in the joint that connects the heel and calf); M
- Patellar tendinopathy (injury to the tissue connecting the kneecap and shin)
- Gluteus medius injuries (hip); F
- Tibial stress fractures (tiny fractures in the shin bone)
- Spinal injuries (back and neck)

Mean weakly hours spent running: 5.4; M = more common in males, F = more common in females.

Some, as indicated, are more significantly common in women, while others show up more often in men. Women also report more sacroiliac injuries, which occur to the sacroiliac joint between the sacrum and the pelvis. Men claim slightly more cases of plantar fasciitis, patellar tendonitis, and Achilles tendinitis.

Most running injuries are caused by repetitive impact and are especially common among individuals with very low BMI (indicating insufficient muscle mass). Notably, across 2,002 runners in the abovementioned study, only 200—ten percent—engaged in weight training in addition to their sport.

female recreational runners over the course of two years. These women were running a minimum of twenty miles (32.2 km) per week. During this two-year period, the number of injured women *outnumbered* the uninjured ones. Of the 144 injured ones, 103 sustained injuries bad enough to require medical attention.

And among the 105 runners who dodged an injury during the observation period, most had been hurt at some point before. Only twenty-one women in the study had never sustained a running injury. They remained, as *New York Times* fitness columnist Gretchen Reynolds put it, "long-term running-injury virgins—the athletic equivalent of unicorns."[171]

If you need medical personnel standing by to participate in your sport, or if escaping injury earns you a comparison to unicorns, it's hard to make the claim that your choice of exercise is keeping you young.

AND THEN THINGS GET REALLY CRAZY

Marathons are just about the worst thing you can do if you're trying to keep your body in youthful condition—that is, with the exception of ultramarathons and triathlons.

In spite of the mounting evidence that excessive cardio is not a good idea, trends continue cropping up that have people logging more miles than ever. Take "streaking"— not running nude, but running consecutively for as many days as possible. To join a streak running club, a person has to run every day,

at least one mile (1.6 k), for 365 consecutive days.[173] From there, individuals compete to see who can accumulate the most years of streaking in a row. Some average up to fourteen miles (22.5 k) per day, interminably.

The question is: Why?

To "meet lifetime mileage goals" is, apparently, one reason. But make no mistake, denying your body a rest just to scratch another mark on a calendar is no longer about health and fitness.

Marathons are just about the worst thing you can do if you're trying to keep your body in youthful condition—that is, with the exception of ultramarathons and triathlons.

Meanwhile, ultramarathoners can be found in Central Park vomiting and hallucinating after completing nine loops in a row—37.2 miles (59.9 km) in roughly nine hours—around the park.[174]

Forget the stupidity of the bloody socks and lost toenails . . . putting your body through the ringer is not only *not* healthy, but it is most certainly dangerous.

"Endurance is the best kind of insurance," Dr. Cooper once prophesized. Clearly, that message was taken too far.

CHASING THE RUNNER'S HIGH

If there were a "fountain of youth," it would be the reduction of distress. Chronic stress takes a toll on the body, damaging hormonal and other chemical balances. In fact, a common trait among people who live long lives is an ability to manage stress—centenarians are often found to have a positive, roll-with-the-punches attitude. Clearly, reducing stress levels is essential both to adding years to your life and life to your years.

While many cite cardio as a stress reliever, there's a dark side, as we've seen: Too much cardio can have the opposite effect.

In 1984, Dr. Henry Solomon dedicated a whole chapter of *The Exercise Myth* to the problematic promise of "runner's high"—the feeling of euphoria, inner peace, and invincibility that many runners claim to experience. This "transcendental" experience usually occurs after running for several miles (11 km).

A group of scientists has even found that runner's high is linked to cannabinoid receptors in the brain—the same ones affected by smoking marijuana.[175] Increased levels of endocannabinoids in the blood after running, as observed by the researchers, led to reduced anxiety and a higher pain tolerance.

So what's the problem? You would think exercise is better for one's health than smoking a joint. The problem is that you might have to increase your volume forever to achieve that runner's high. Consider the "hedonic treadmill," which means that gradually, our emotional response to a pleasant stimulus wears off, if the stimulus stays constant.[176] This may be one reason that ultramarathoners continually set the bar higher.

(Geez, does that sound familiar? It's like any other addiction!)

That "cloud nine" feeling might subside when your knees are crunchy and your hormones are out of whack from decades of running.

"The belief that the reward of a high surpasses the punishment required to attain it means you must push yourself ever harder, beyond the boundaries of everyday risk, and the limits of prudence," Solomon wrote. "It demands that you suspend awareness of symptoms, of warning signals of fatigue and pain. The belief plummets you toward danger." That "cloud nine" feeling might subside when your knees are crunchy and your hormones are out of whack from decades of running.

Rather than putting unhealthy stress on the body in pursuit of psychological benefits, there are other, safer, ways to get an exercise endorphin boost. A regimen with lots of variety is one way, and it can help limit overuse injuries. (Doing the same thing over and over again, as many do in a cardio routine, is also a great way to feel old!) Another way is a workout that requires focus. Psychologists have found that engagement in what we're doing, as opposed to multitasking, leads to a "flow" state that most people find deeply rewarding and motivating. Being present and focused can help you avoid injury, too.

If you truly enjoy cardio, then it's fine to keep it up at low levels, as long as you're not overzealous to the point of reversing the benefits—putting too much physical stress on the body, opening yourself up to injuries, or diminishing the protective health benefits of exercise, as Solomon warned.

Yet, a lot of people don't enjoy their cardio routine. It's evident in the TV, books, magazines, and other things many use to distract themselves.

There are a number of activities that can relieve psychological stress. Strength training, dog walks, reading, meditation, and helping others—these are what do it for me. Maybe you'll find it in time with family and friends, hobbies, work you enjoy—all great stress relievers. So is an exercise regimen that allows you time for those things.

SO WHAT ABOUT PLAIN OLD GYM CARDIO?

Up to now we've been looking at injuries and other dangers of extreme cardio exercise. Surely it's a different story with average cardio workouts . . . right?

Not necessarily. Though the average jogger is less likely to pass out in a bush after seeing stars, injuries are still a common occurrence. That's because many less-experienced runners have improper technique and insufficient conditioning.[177]

A recent meta-analysis in the journal *Sports Medicine* found higher injury rates in recreational runners than ultramarathoners and *significantly* higher injury rates in novice runners.[178] While recreational runners suffered 7.7 injuries per 1,000 running hours (and ultramarathoners, 7.2 injuries), novice runners sustained 17.8—more than double! For a novice runner, that could mean one injury for every fifty-six hours of running.

When starting out, some runners and joggers do too much too soon, leading to acute injuries. It comes back to the belief that it's convenient and natural and anyone can do it.

Yet, as we just saw, seasoned athletes are just as likely to sustain injuries, including the chronic overuse kind that will really make you feel old before your time.

There are running guides to help people avoid injury, but most everyday runners and joggers aren't reading them. Dr. Nicholas Romanov, in his book *The Running Revolution*, admits that about two-thirds of runners are injured every year. Like many of today's running evangelists, he claims humans were "born to run." It makes you wonder, if humans were "born to run," shouldn't we have a better sense of how to avoid injury while doing it?

Tallying up the injuries, it doesn't seem as though humans were optimally built for running. In fact, the human body was probably not designed for long, arduous, repetitive activity of any kind. People wind up injured from popular cardio classes all the time, for many of the same reasons.

Take spinning. A medical center in Korea recently reported an increase in people showing up with injuries after attending their first spin class.[179] Following a rigorous bout of indoor cycling, eleven women arrived at the emergency room complaining of thigh soreness, extreme fatigue, and brown urine. These women were diagnosed with rhabdomyolysis, a potentially serious condition wherein muscle fibers are broken down and their content is released into the blood, hence the brown urine.[180] The women were treated with aggressive intravenous fluid and bed rest. Luckily for them, it wasn't more serious.

Other emergency rooms have filed similar reports and expressed concern about the increasing popularity of spin classes.[181] According to the United States National Library of Medicine, spinning, along with marathon running, military training, and other highly strenuous activities, are all common causes of rhabdomyolysis. When treated immediately, athletes with milder forms of the condition can recover within a few weeks. Long term, it can cause kidney damage.

Such repercussions of extreme exertion aren't limited to cardio, of course; they can occur with just about any form of intense physical activity (CrossFit comes to mind). Any exercise poses risks if you're overdoing

it, but the injury numbers are astronomically higher with aerobic exercise, in part because it is performed for longer—sometimes extremely long—durations.

Another reason might be that extreme-endurance exercise is often performed in a herd, where people may be more likely to push themselves beyond what is comfortable or safe. Think about an intense spin class, with the music blaring and the instructor shouting at you to push harder, or a marathon, with people cheering you on from the sidelines.

The only population that keeps my chiropractor friends busier than CrossFit attendees is runners.

I've worked with physiotherapists so addicted to spinning that they couldn't walk properly and marathon runners that could only shuffle through a marathon because their body was so beat up and they refused to take time off.

The only population that keeps my chiropractor friends busier than CrossFit attendees is runners. Many runners are addicted to their workouts, either because they experience that runner's high or because they become fixated on burning a certain amount of calories per day, and this leads to overdoing it.

HORMONAL CHANGES IN MEN AND WOMEN

Beyond obvious injuries and overexertion, a high volume of cardio can lead to hormonal changes in the body. These can have negative consequences over time, from making weight loss harder to hindering reproductive function in both men and women.

One major change is an increase in the hormone cortisol. Cortisol levels fluctuate in response to stress. A growing body of research shows increased levels of cortisol in the blood, saliva, and hair of endurance athletes, signaling chronic physical or psychological stress.

A 2012 study compared amateur male and female endurance athletes to a control group of regular exercisers.[182] The 300 endurance athletes—mostly long-distance runners, cyclists, and triathletes—had significantly higher cortisol levels than the average exercisers who did light jogging or exercise at the gym.

"During acute stress," the study authors explained, "the metabolic, behavioral, cognitive, and immunological effects of cortisol fulfill adaptive functions helping the organism deal with the present challenge or threat to homeostasis."

Is this a bad thing? Well, some experts believe that if cortisol levels return to normal within a few days, there's nothing to worry about. However, the researchers behind the 2012 study think we have reason to be concerned. They concluded that, "long-term alterations in cortisol release may have detrimental effects on health," because chronically increased cortisol levels "may be a potential contributing factor in the disease pathway."

Leptin is another hormone affected by long bouts of exercise. Leptin is secreted by the pituitary gland and regulates, among many things, appetite, reproductive function, and body weight.[183] In a study of female athletes on a college rowing team, researchers observed decreased leptin concentrations in ten of the seventeen women on a rigorous training schedule.[184] These women were identified as "responders," and their bodies showed an attempt to adapt to the intense training— rowing, running, or weight lifting, every day for twenty weeks.

In this study, the effect—decreased levels of leptin—was significant after controlling for confounding factors like differences in training level and body composition. Further, these women had no prior endocrine system problems. Scientists guess the response occurs in an effort to save energy during high caloric expenditure (recall Pontzer's plateau, see page 71).

But the adaptation may not be harmless. The leptin changes in the just-referenced study were observed at rest, and the disruptions persisted even after the intense training period was over. The researchers suggested that such disruptions could impair proper functioning of the neuroendocrine system, including energy metabolism and growth development.

THE FEMALE ATHLETE TRIAD

Back in college, I remember going to the house of a girlfriend who lived with what I called exercise addicts. These women would do hours of cardio, then come home and eat boxes of cereal, and do it all over again the next day. Some researchers refer to this as exercise bulimia.

Cardio seems to foster an "eat it, burn it" weight loss mentality more than any other activity. In fact, a condition called the female athlete triad is strongly connected to excessive cardio and body image disorders.[185]

The potential for overdoing it with endurance *exercise is particularly strong, maybe because of the myth that more cardio is better, as well as the wild popularity of marathons and other competitive endurance events.*

The "Triad" is a group of interrelated conditions—amenorrhea (absence of menstruation), brittle bones, and energy deficiency—that can harm reproductive health and increase the risk of breaking bones and developing osteoporosis. According to the American College of Sports Medicine, it can even be fatal.[186] The trio of complications is caused by insufficient nutrition relative to exertion (the opposite problem of the marathoners you'll meet in chapter 6). Sometimes, it stems from trying to achieve unrealistic thinness to compete in one's sport or out of an obsession with burning off every calorie a person eats. It can also arise from exercise addiction or the pursuit of a strenuous athletic goal.

An intensive exercise regimen can have detrimental effects on reproductive function, even if you do have proper nutrition. Some studies show an association with disruption of ovarian function, despite sufficient calorie intake.[187]

The potential for overdoing it with *endurance* exercise is particularly strong, maybe because of the myth that more cardio is better, as well as the wild popularity of marathons and other competitive endurance events.

LOWER TESTOSTERONE IN MEN

In 2016, Ryan Hall, the fastest American distance runner in history, decided to throw in the towel on the U.S. Olympic marathon trials—and marathons altogether—because of chronic low testosterone and extreme fatigue.[188] "It felt like I was melting into the ground," Hall told *Runner's World*.[189]

Hall had spent the past four years trying to correct the health condition. He worked with doctors and coaches and experimented with diet and his training program. "At the end of the day, it all just led back to the same place, which was extreme fatigue," he said. At one point Hall could no longer even finish a thirty-minute run.

After cutting way back on his running, down to a few half-hour runs a week, Hall picked up weight training instead and managed to put on a lot of muscle in a short amount of time—which he said not only felt great, but also helped increase his testosterone levels.

Several studies have linked endurance exercise with persistent low resting levels of testosterone in men. Yet researchers aren't entirely sure why. One study indicates it might be stress related; the scientists pinpointed an inverse relationship between lower total testosterone levels and increased cortisol, triggered by prolonged strenuous endurance exercise.[190] "Regardless of the potential mechanism, to our knowledge, the present study is the first to demonstrate that exercise-induced cortisol changes show a negative relationship with subsequent circulating testosterone levels," the authors concluded. However, they noted that because of the study design, they could only make correlational inferences about the increased cortisol and decreased testosterone.

CARDIAC OVERUSE INJURY AND WHAT WE CAN LEARN FROM PHEIDIPPIDES

And then there is the potential for cardiovascular damage. Recall from chapter 3 the running tipping point after which all heart health bets are essentially off (see page 53).

In the Copenhagen City Heart Study, the longevity benefits vanished in people running twenty miles (32.2 km) or more per week.[191] Cardiologist James O'Keefe and his colleagues also noted that chronic exercise doses get riskier with age, especially after age forty-five or fifty.

O'Keefe, currently at Saint Luke's Mid America Heart Institute, once won the largest sprint distance triathlon in Kansas City. But he gave up on extreme endurance exercise after weighing the benefits of athletic achievement against the drawbacks: mounting evidence of potential heart damage and his own sense that it was aging him prematurely.[192]

We all know the Olympic tale of Pheidippides, the courier who, in 490 B.C.E., ran for two days to Athens to deliver news of a victory against the Persians in the Battle of Marathon. According to legend, he then died on the spot. While this story is surely folklore, people still want to test fate.

Today, some actually refer to the aftermath of cardiac overuse injury—which can include dangerous rhythmic abnormalities, fibrosis and scarring of the myocardium, and accelerated coronary atherosclerosis—as Pheidippides cardiomyopathy.

Granted, risk of sudden death during a marathon is moderately low (0.8 to 2 per 100,000 people), and it isn't always caused by cardiac arrest. Triathletes—who have a comparable risk of dying mid race (1.5 deaths in 100,000)—are most likely to kick the bucket during the swimming portion.[193] The most common cause is drowning, as well as sudden cardiac death and blunt trauma.

Many still kid themselves that extreme exercise is keeping them young. It isn't easy to let go of long-held beliefs about what we should be doing for our health. But even Dr. Cooper changed his mind in light of evolving research. He now advises that fifteen to twenty miles (24.1 to 32.2 km) a week is the threshold for achieving health benefits.[194] Others might say, after browsing the small sampling of evidence in this chapter, that the threshold is lower.

Dr. Schnohr, who is on the Copenhagen City Heart Study team at Frederiksberg Hospital in Denmark, recommends that joggers cap their regimen at one and a half or two hours of low- to moderate-intensity jogging per week.[195] That probably won't lead to fat loss or muscle gain, and it could still take a toll on your knees. For those who love running, however, staying on the conservative side is surely better.

EFFECTS OF THE ENVIRONMENT

Most of America's sixty-five million runners and joggers exercise outside.[196] In 2013, 57.6 million people were running, walking, or trail running outdoors on a regular basis.[197] A close second, 46.6 million Americans reported road and mountain biking as the other top activity.

It's a natural impulse to get outside and move your body. In fact, many might consider going for a jog as a healthy way to be out of doors and enjoy some fresh air. Getting out of the house, away from the office, and into some sunshine (with sunblock, of course) should be a great stress reliever.

But for those who spend hours and hours doing cardio outside, it can increase cellular aging that shows up as skin cancer, as well as increase breathing of pollutants and breakdown of healthy joints. (Pavement and concrete are nightmares on the joints.)[198]

Runners have good reason to be concerned about air quality, given the amount of carbon monoxide belched from exhaust pipes on a daily basis. Particularly troubling is the extreme popularity of endurance races in highly polluted cities, such as Los Angeles and New York City, where annual races see up to 50,000 entrants every year.

Skin cancer is an even greater concern. Cumulative sun damage can silently increase cancer risk—ironically, while people are out running for their health. Endurance athletes face a heightened risk of malignant melanoma and non-melanoma skin cancer, studies show. Among one observation of marathoners with malignant melanoma, researchers noted that over a ten-year span these runners wore shorts and shirts that exposed their backs and/or extremities more than 90 percent of the time.[199] Only 56.2 percent reported regularly using sunscreen.

GOOD STRESS VERSUS BAD STRESS

In a way, exercise is effective *because* it puts stress on the body. That's the whole point: It forces the body out of its comfort zone and makes it expend extra energy, and it breaks down muscle fibers so the body will build them up even stronger.

But there is a difference between positive stress (eustress) and unhealthy stress (distress). Too much physical stress falls into the second category. Overtraining is what happens in an overstressed body pushed too hard or not given sufficient recovery time. Overtraining causes not just physical, but also psychological, stress.

This is something all exercisers have to be cautious of. Intense activities stress the body; however, short burst exercise can rarely be sustained for long durations, which may be why people are less likely to overdo it (in addition to the fact that you need less of it for significant results, as we saw in chapter 4). It's the same with strength training. It's important to stick with a program that starts slowly and progressively and listen to your body.

The great Jack LaLanne, one of the first people to promote weight lifting for general fitness, said, "Like wine, you should be able to improve with age." I completely agree. One of the big promises of cardio—starting with the invention of aerobics and the running trend in the 1960s—is that it would help us look and feel younger. But despite some clear short-term benefits, the long-term effect appears to be negative for many people.

The side effects discussed in this chapter are in addition to the *major* potential pitfalls of cardio: gaining weight, losing muscle, and eating poorly (more on that in the next chapter), all of which can definitely have you feeling older than your years!

Overtraining is what happens in an overstressed body pushed too hard or not given sufficient recovery time.

I'm happy to report that Catherine is no longer afraid of going to the grocery store on Senior Discount Tuesday. Being mistaken for a senior at forty-four was the last straw, causing her to quit her cardio-based regimen and take up my program of interval and metabolic resistance training, combined with improved nutrition. Actually, as you'll see in chapter 7, strength training is probably the best thing you can do to stay young after age forty. After just twelve weeks of her new regimen, Catherine had already dropped fourteen pounds (6.4 kg) and lost inches everywhere, especially her waist. More important . . . she felt and looked fifteen years younger.

Side note: At one point Catherine tried switching back to her Zumba regimen, but when the pounds started creeping back on, she quit for good!

WHAT YOU NEED TO KNOW

- Exercise is supposed to keep us young, preventing health problems from the minor (creaky knees, aching backs, and "muffin tops") to the major (cancer, diabetes, osteoporosis, and heart disease). Yet, excessive cardio can have the opposite effect, making these problems worse.

- Cardio is linked with hormone changes that make muscle gain and weight loss harder. In high amounts, it can also negatively affect the male and female reproductive endocrine systems.

- For those who exercise outside for long periods, cardio might really make you feel older: It can increase cellular aging that shows up as skin cancer, increase the breathing of pollutants, and contribute to the breakdown of healthy joints.

- Up to 90 percent of runners sustain injuries, including strain on the knees, stress fractures, and ankle sprains. The repetitive pounding on joints can be especially harmful if you're heavy or overweight.

On average,
people over-estimate
the number
of calories burned
during a 25-minute
treadmill walk
by 72%.

6

1 MILE ≠ 1 CUPCAKE

AS THEY LIMPED across the finish line of the New York City Marathon, three women—coming in well after the last official recorded time—were dreaming up their reward meals. "I don't know how many calories I've burned," one of them told a reporter, "but I'm going to do my damnedest to put them back in."[200]

Another shared some good news: She had burned the equivalent of twenty-four cupcakes during their 26.2-mile (42.2 km) schlep around the city. They had the green light to gorge, she told her friends. Heck, they could have indulged in a cupcake at every mile (1.6 km) marker!

It's not hard to imagine that every runner who crossed the finish line that day had some variation of the same thought running through their heads.

I just earned a whole pizza and a side of bread sticks!

I just bought myself the biggest hot fudge sundae of my life!

I can eat anything I want!

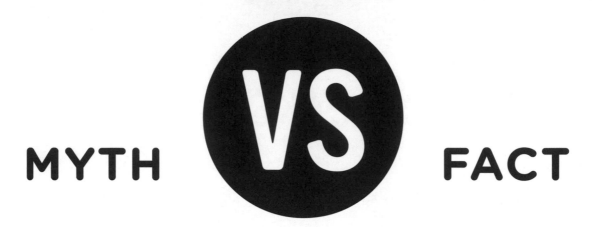

MYTH VS FACT

MYTH	FACT
Fat loss is a simple "calories in, calories out" equation.	The relationship between food, exercise, and body composition is much more complex.
If the cardio machine says you burned 300 calories, your exercise regimen is working.	Calorie burn counters on exercise machines are significantly inaccurate. What's more, long cardio workouts may cause you to conserve calories elsewhere throughout your day.
Many endurance exercisers are skinny, which proves cardio is good for staying slim.	Some endurance exercisers are "skinny fat," meaning they have a small frame but not a lot of muscle mass.
If you exercise regularly, you can eat whatever you want.	You can't out-exercise a bad diet! We're notoriously bad at balancing calories "earned" with calories burned. Besides, not all calories are created equal.

Lengthy exercise sessions have a funny way of playing tricks on the mind. And it doesn't just happen to marathoners. Hour-long treadmill sessions send people running for the buffet line, too. People often think they're outpacing their caloric intake, but, as it turns out, we're generally pretty bad at calorie math. In this chapter, you'll find out why exercise, and cardio in particular, rarely delivers the calorie burn mileage you expect. There are three major reasons:

1. We eat more calories than we think.

2. We burn fewer calories than we think.

3. We move less outside the gym.

Let's consider each reason.

REASON 1: WE EAT MORE CALORIES THAN WE THINK

According to "mindless eating" guru Dr. Brian Wansink, the average person *under* estimates daily caloric intake by about 20 percent.[201] If you're overweight, it's closer to 30 to 40 percent.

That means if you think you're eating 2,000 calories a day, it could actually be closer to 2,500 . . . or more. If that sounds shocking, let's check the marathoner's cupcake math.

On average, a person burns one hundred calories running one mile (1.6 k).[202] So:

1 mile (1.6 k) = 100 calories, but

1 cupcake = 300 calories (according to Google)

As you can see, that's not exactly one cupcake per mile (1.6 k) marker. So what would have happened if this runner treated herself to a cupcake for every mile she ran during the marathon?

Calories eaten: 26 cupcakes ✕ 300 calories = 7,800

Calories burned: 26.2 miles (42.2 km) ✕ 100 calories = 2,620

Estimated calorie surplus: 5,180!

A marathoner burns an extra day of calories in a race, yet so many use this as an excuse to feast and gorge. And I can't say I blame them: If you're exercising for nine miserable hours, which is how long it took those three women to finish the marathon, then it certainly seems like you *should* be able to eat anything you want—with no guilt.

But nature isn't so generous.

If you have the same calorie (mis)counting mentality during months and months of marathon training, it's going to spell trouble. And it's not just a marathon mindset.

Every year my friend has a Super Bowl party. More than seventy-five personal trainers, nutritionists, and physiotherapists gather in his backyard in southern Florida to watch the big game . . . and more importantly, to binge eat food they otherwise avoid all year long.

It's a ridiculous scene. Dozens of them eat themselves into immobility, and many of them complain about how painful their stomachs feel. They also brag about how they fasted and did excessive amounts of cardio during the day to make up for it.

They are as foolish as any client I've ever worked with. They know better! They know that the calories in a dozen chicken wings, four slices of pizza, six chocolate cookies, and bowl of ice cream far exceed what they could burn off in even a literal marathon training session—and yet they still justify their binge eating through exercise.

It's not a battle you can ever win, especially on Super Bowl Sunday.

We all know (I hope) that "a calorie isn't a calorie." In other words, a 400-calorie Vanilla Buttercream cupcake from Starbucks isn't the nutrition equivalent of a 400-calorie quinoa salad. And high-fat, high-sugar foods are going to have a negative effect on your body no matter how much penance you pay in the gym.

That said, we usually get the "calories *burned*" math wrong, too.

REASON 2: WE BURN FEWER CALORIES THAN WE THINK

A recent study found that, after walking on a treadmill at a vigorous pace for twenty-five minutes, people overestimated calories burned by 72 percent.[203] The overweight participants inflated their estimated calorie burn the most. It's just one more reason you can't out-train a bad diet.

To illustrate the point, I recently filmed a YouTube video wherein I tried to outrun . . . pizza.[204] Okay, I ran while my friend, nutritionist Brad Pilon, stood next to the treadmill and packed away the pizza, finishing a giant slice and a soda in three minutes while I ran as fast as I could for the same amount of time. The goal was to see whether three minutes of pleasure equated to the same amount of pain—since that's how we usually do the calorie math in our heads, right?

I was running 10.5 miles (16.9 k) per hour, which is faster than *most* people are going to run as self-punishment for yesterday's splurge. But running my heart out was no match for the 800 calories Brad managed to gulp down in the same timeframe that I burned . . . wait for it . . . forty calories.

The point I hope you take away from this is one long session at the "cardio confessional" does not make up for one binge-eating session. It's not even close.

And don't let the calorie-burn counters fool you. . . . These days, the screen on almost every cardio machine at the gym, from stationary bikes and stair-steppers to rowing machines and ellipticals, will tell you how many calories you're burning during your workout.

Unfortunately, those tallies are highly inaccurate.

One study found elliptical machines to be the *least*-accurate cardio machine at the gym.[205] It was especially inaccurate—inflating reported calorie burn—in women and when exercising at higher intensities.

Sheesh. It makes me wonder if I even burned that measly forty calories on the treadmill during my "pizza race!"

One long session at the "cardio confessional" does not make up for one binge-eating session. It's not even close.

It gets worse. Some machines calculate your gross, instead of net, energy expenditure, which means the output includes your resting metabolic rate . . . or how many calories you'd be burning if you were just sitting on the couch.[206]

Meanwhile, if you lean on the handrails of a stair-stepper or treadmill, that machine doesn't know it, so it will overestimate your expenditure, adding to the already overinflated numbers.

Some cardio machine manufacturers are even considering screen enhancements, such as simulations of how many calories a user is burning and what food it equates to.[207] I can't imagine anything more disastrous: distract exercisers from being fully engaged in their workout, lie to them about how many calories they're burning, and show them pictures of food they can eat after as a reward for all that hard work they supposedly did!

TREAT-FUELED TREADMILL SESSIONS

Add another report to the pile. Simone Dohle and Brian Wansink published research in the *Journal of Physical Activity and Health* supporting the theory that exercisers don't lose weight because they increase their caloric intake after exercise.[208]

After conducting focus groups with twenty-seven people who exercised one to five hours a week, post-exercise food rewards emerged as a common theme: "Participants reported that when they were active, they lost their guilt about unhealthy food choices or the amount of food they ate."

But is it just bad calorie math, like we saw before? No. It's actually more complicated because the cardio workouts led people to different attitudes about food and how much they actually needed to refuel after a normal workout. They were also more likely to succumb to cravings, for physiological reasons (some subjects reported unusually strong hunger an hour after their workouts) and because of the "treat" mentality.

Men in one study increased carbohydrate intake during a long-term running program.[209] In another, high-intensity treadmill walking caused exercisers to scarf more at a lunch buffet following their workouts than they did on non-exercise days.[210] (Notably, they also ate more than the non-exercising control group.)

In a published review of the literature on exercise and food intake, researchers Sonya

Elder and Susan Roberts concluded that, "exercised individuals may feel less restraint due to a sense of physical accomplishment, and may choose foods normally viewed as unhealthy, such as foods high in sugar or fat."[211]

I've watched people consuming sugary energy drinks during a thirty-minute elliptical session or "carb loading" after a sixty-minute bike ride or treadmill session. Both of which are totally unnecessary for the majority of everyday exercisers! But sometimes people aren't even aware they're doing it.

Some people serve themselves more food just thinking *of exercise.*[216] *It's the "I've earned it" mentality.*

While some exercisers use cardio to justify extra calories, others mindlessly answer to heightened cravings.[212–213] Research has found that people eat as much as 44 percent more dessert after exercise and 32 percent fewer vegetables than they normally would.[214] Apparently, it's not uncommon for people to start knocking back extra beers thanks to exercise.[215]

Even more horrifying: some people serve themselves more food just *thinking* of exercise.[216] It's the "I've earned it" mentality. Whether consciously or unconsciously, exercisers feel they deserve a reward. And the more boring and miserable the workout, the more likely you are to do it.[217]

That brings us to why marathons might actually be the worst appetite offender of all.

WHY SOME MARATHONERS ARE FATTER AT THE FINISH LINE

Marathons. Many a recreational runner sets her heart on this big goal and expects to lose weight and get in shape in the training process. Millions of individuals sacrifice sleep and weekends to run for hours on end. And yet, from a fat loss perspective, the payoff is often meager. Sometimes, it's even abysmal.

After eighteen months of running miles and miles on most days of the week, women in one study didn't lose any weight at all. In other marathon training studies, participants have either lost a mere handful of pounds (again, usually men) or gained weight.

Researchers at Tufts University were curious.[218] "Despite conventional wisdom, a majority of runners do not lose body weight while training for a marathon," they wrote. So they monitored sixty-four men and women who were training to run a springtime marathon.

On average, the runners logged 24.5 miles (39.4 k) a week spread across four days. Three months later, when it was time for check-in, the mean body mass index of the group was unchanged. Most of them (78 percent) came out at the same weight as when they started, while 11 percent lost weight and 11 percent gained it. Of those who added pounds, nearly all were women.

They were baffled . . . until they examined the food logs. Half the men and three-quarters of the women reported an increase in calories. The researchers had their answer about marathons and meager weight loss: "It appears that an increase in caloric intake, especially in females, plays an important role in this result."

In another study out of the Netherlands, sixteen men and sixteen women, ages twenty-eight to forty-one, trained to run a half marathon.[219] The results were the same. Over the course of forty weeks, men managed to shed a few pounds of fat, but the women's results were only half that of the men's. The researchers concluded that women tend to compensate for increased energy expenditure by eating more. Whereas men's energy intake tended to drop between week 20 and week 40, women's energy intake increased during that timeframe. The more they ran, the more they gobbled up extra calories unknowingly.

Similarly, Janssen and colleagues found that an eighteen-month marathon-training period left men a little lighter (5.3 pounds [2.4 kg], on average), while no change in body composition was observed in women.[220]

We're talking running miles and miles a day: no weight change for the women and a measly five pounds (2.3 kg) for the guys.

That moment of shock is familiar to many people after training for their first marathon. It might even be one you've experienced!

REASON 3: WE MOVE LESS OUTSIDE THE GYM

More cardio, more couch time? Even if you vow to keep your calories in check, you might still get less calorie burn than you're expecting from your cardio routine. Researchers have found it can lead to less physical activity outside the gym.

It comes back to Pontzer's plateau from chapter 4 (see page 71). Dr. Pontzer and his team found that long bouts of exercise led people to compensate—basically, to recoup energy, or calories—in a number of ways. A survival mechanism, perhaps . . . but it's not particularly helpful when you're trying to lose weight.

In addition to eating more calories, they noticed other compensatory mechanisms. Physiologically, the body can adapt and use less energy to do the same activity, which means lower calorie burn. That's *on top* of the muscle-loss-induced decline in metabolism that can happen with excessive cardio and no strength training.

But compensation can also be behavioral and unconscious, Pontzer and his team explained—"sitting instead of standing, or fidgeting less."[221] Echoing their finding, a new study out of the University of South Carolina found that subjects who did aerobic exercise became *less* active in daily life, while strength training had the opposite effect.[222]

In addition to sitting instead of standing, the compensation effect can also take the form

DON'T BE FOOLED BY SKINNY RUNNERS

We've seen dozens of studies that show cardio to be less effective for fat loss than HIIT and strength training. We've also seen that it's common for marathon runners to *gain* weight during training.

I know what you're thinking. *What about all those thin runners I see pounding the pavement?*

Before you use them as your fitness models, consider this:

1. It's possible they really are keeping their body fat percentage low with cardio. Some people do. They can thank their genes, I guess. (And they are mostly, shock and horror, young men with the world's best hormonal milieu on their side. And time. Plenty of time to exercise for hours a day.)

2. It's possible they're skinny fat—actually, this is the more likely answer, especially if they're out there running circles around the park for an hour every day. They may look fine from a distance, but under those jogging suits they're probably flabby and weak due to muscle loss from years (or even just months) of endurance exercise with no strength training.

3. And there's a third possibility: self-selection bias. A number of studies have detected that endurance cardio tends to attract slimmer people. In a large observational study across seven to ten years, more than 70 percent of walkers had a low BMI prior to starting their program.[224] In another study of walking and running distances, leaner participants at the outset tended to exercise faster and go further, while fatter ones opted for the shorter route.[225] Perhaps the overweight find it uncomfortable to exercise for long durations, the researchers noted.

of choosing the elevator instead of climbing the stairs or grabbing the shuttle instead of walking. By the end of the sixteen-week study, the aerobic exercisers had decreased their physical activity outside the gym not only on exercise days, but also on non-workout days and weekends, too.

Subjects who did aerobic exercise became less active in daily life, while strength training had the opposite effect.[222]

"Resistance exercise, on the other hand, appears to facilitate non-exercise [physical activity]," the study authors concluded, "particularly on non-exercise days, which may lead to more sustainable adaptations in response to an exercise program."

There's no shortage of research telling us that a daily workout won't save us if we're plunked in a chair the rest of the time.[223] Exercise that motivates us to stay active outside the gym is the better choice. It's better for functional fitness, maintaining metabolism and muscle, and reaping the cumulative health benefits of exercise over the lifespan.

Looking at Figures 6.1 and 6.2, which show changes in daily activity in response to aerobic and strength programs, you see that, despite increasing energy expenditure on workout days by week 16, the *aerobics* group (Fig. 6.1) hadn't become much more active the rest of the week. Conversely, the *resistance* group (Fig. 6.2) increased energy expenditure on both workout days *and* non-workout days and weekends. They spent more time on moderate to vigorous activity than they did before and burned more calories than the aerobic exercisers did on non-workout days.

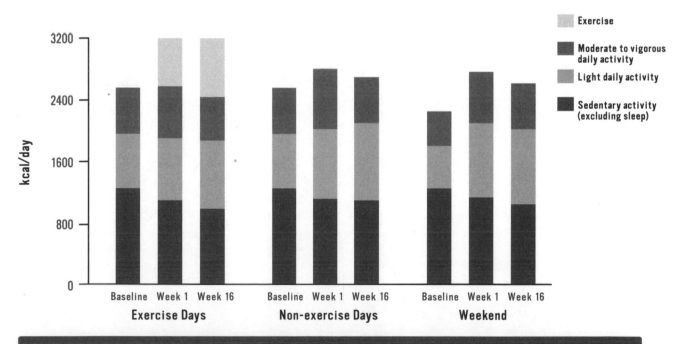

AEROBIC EXERCISERS

Figure 6.1: Despite increasing energy expenditure on workout days, the aerobics group did not become much more active the rest of the week.

ONE STEP FORWARD, TWO STEPS BACK

People often forget why they started exercising in the first place—to create a calorie deficit, lose fat, and get healthy. Instead, they start seeing their workouts as a way to buy extra junk-food splurges. I had one client who confessed to a past gym ritual (which she probably thought was uncommon): swinging by McDonald's for a burger after her forty-five-minute sessions on the elliptical. It had become her routine, three times a week, all through her college years.

> *Exercise that motivates us to stay active outside the gym is the better choice.*

We're talking 410 calories in a Quarter Pounder with cheese (let's hope she didn't get the 710-calorie Double Quarter Pounder). And I guarantee she didn't burn that doing forty-five minutes of low-intensity cardio. She probably burned 250 calories, at best . . . if she was working hard.

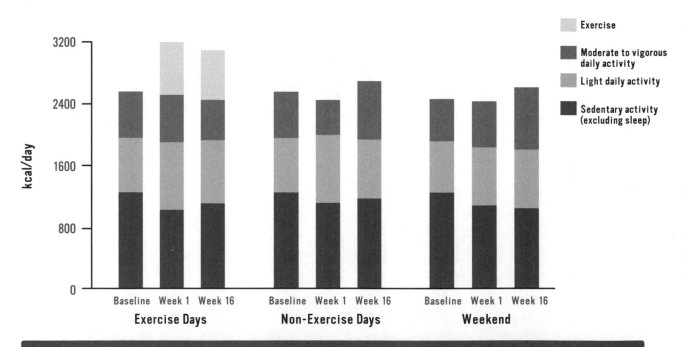

RESISTANCE EXERCISERS
Figure 6.2: The resistance group increased energy expenditure on both workout days and non-workout days and weekends.

COMPENSATION 101

Energy expenditure ceiling: Remember Dr. Pontzer's studies, where people's daily "energy costs" were about the same, whether they did a ton of walking or barely any at all (see page 71)? It revealed a daily calorie-burn threshold or "ceiling" that appears to be built-in with humans.

Behavioral compensation effect: Engaging in lots of exercise can lead people to compensate to stay within the energy expenditure (EE) threshold. One way is with food and drink. In Pontzer's (and other) studies, people who moved more ate more, even when they didn't need to.

Physiological compensation effect: The body also finds sneaky ways to expend less energy, becoming more efficient and, "adapting to high levels of habitual physical activity," Pontzer explains. If you reach the EE threshold during exercise, you might become less physically active during non-exercise times. That's why hours of steady-state cardio can lead to a declining rate of energy expenditure—something the cardio machines won't pick up!

Why non-cardio might be exempt: Studies showing the compensation effect almost always have a common denominator—people doing steady-state cardio. Research suggests that HIIT has a lower energy cost despite producing better fat loss.[226] Similarly, strength training has a lower energy expenditure compared with cardio workouts of the same duration. Thus, you're less likely to hit your energy expenditure ceiling and trigger a rebound effect.

At the same time, HIIT and resistance exercise produce positive effects on fat loss over the long term, despite lower energy expenditure, due to improvements to metabolism. With regard to physiological adaptation, putting *turbulence* on the body, (see page 79), appears to help prevent the body from getting more efficient (i.e., burning fewer calories) doing the same activity.

Using exercise to justify a fast-food splurge is just about the worst thing you can do. Fast food has been pegged as the culprit behind most accidental calorie overconsumption.[227-228]

Thankfully, that woman eventually wised up and ditched both the burgers and the elliptical machine—though not before a couple years of genuine confusion about why she wasn't getting the results she wanted at the gym.

It's like rewards cards. You watch the points rack up and tell yourself you're saving all that money. In the end, you spend *way* more money than you would have otherwise just because you have the points. If the cardio machine tells you you're burning a burger's worth of calories, you're more likely to say, "What the heck!" and indulge.

And then there's the other cardio camp: the people who believe they should do cardio but hate it. They feel as though they need a reward to atone for the pain of another hour-long treadmill session. Or they think marathon races should have cupcakes at every mile marker.

A shorter, more mentally engaging workout can save you the trouble of a pain-and-reward cycle. In fact, Dr. Wansink says choosing a workout you *enjoy* is one of the best ways to avoid excessive exercise-induced calorie compensation.[229]

The big lesson: Cardio leads to overeating in two ways. First, the mental justification shown by the trainers at the Super Bowl party, who should know better. And also physiologically, on a smaller scale, in the phenomenon described by Dr. Pontzer and others.

I find both strength training and interval training do the opposite to my appetite, and many others feel the same way after a difficult resistance training session. Even if you were slightly hungry before, your liver releases a lot of glucose into the blood during intense exercise (to fuel it), and thus your blood sugar stabilizes. And because of the increase in blood lactate from intervals and short burst resistance training, you tend to have a reduction in appetite for an hour after exercise.

Also, short burst exercise increases adrenaline (epinephrine), a hormone in the flight-or-fight stress response. As most people know,

when under periods of acute stress, they don't feel like eating.

For those who want to gain muscle weight, you often have to force feed yourself in that time if you need the extra calories.

FIND A WORKOUT THAT WORKS WITH YOU

One of the most important aspects of exercise is how it affects your body and behavior when you're *not* exercising. While building muscle and burning calories are important, many of the benefits—or drawbacks—take place *outside the gym*. That includes how exercise affects your motivation, your metabolism, your energy levels throughout the day, your mental well-being, and, perhaps most important, your food habits.

I have never had a client who justified a calorie binge with a promise to lift weights the next day to make up for it. And in the studies mentioned above, people were doing steady-state exercise. But even if they studied calorie compensation after strength training or short burst workouts, I don't think you'd see the problem as much. I haven't.

So, what is it about cardio? For one, it's the machine calorie counters, which encourage this kind of "calorie in, calorie out" thinking.

Two, it's the long duration and monotony of most cardio activities, especially those done on machines. It leads people to think—consciously or unconsciously—they've earned a treat for suffering through it. Heck, it's the only way some people can bring themselves to suffer through the monotony . . . planning a reward in advance for the punishment! It's like bribing your six-year-old with candy to stay quiet in church (which is what my mom did to get me to behave).

Of course you'll have to be conscious of your eating habits no matter what type of exercise you do (that's where chapter 9 comes in). But there are some extra forces working against you with long cardio. It's better to have your workouts working with you than against you!

WHAT YOU NEED TO KNOW

- People underestimate the number of calories they consume by up to 30 to 40 percent. We also tend to overestimate the amount of calories we burn during workouts and faulty machine counters don't help.

- Cardio leads some people to crave and justify desserts and fast food, leaving their waistlines even wider than if they'd skipped the workout altogether!

- Research suggests that women are even more likely to compensate for increased energy expenditure by eating more.

Sedentary adults lose 3 to 8% of muscle mass per decade.

7

STRENGTH TRAINING:
THE NEW RUNNING FOR THE OVER-FORTIES

YOU DUTIFULLY GO to your annual check-up, and your doctor pats you on the back for doing your daily cardio and sends you on your way. Never mind that since you turned forty you've been getting fatter, your knees hurt, and your blood pressure measurements are nowhere near as good as they should be considering all the hours you spend pounding the pavement.

You're meeting the standard physical activity recommendation and that's what matters, right?

Well, maybe I just eat too much, you think. *That must be the reason I'm gaining five pounds (2.3 kg) a year.* So you go on a diet.

That doesn't really help. You lose a few pounds, but you still feel flabby. So you decide to up your daily cardio. Instead of forty-five minutes a day, you clock an hour.

Despite your efforts, over time, your waistline expands. Your bottom sags. Your arms and legs press at the seams of your clothing. What happened? I'll hazard a guess.

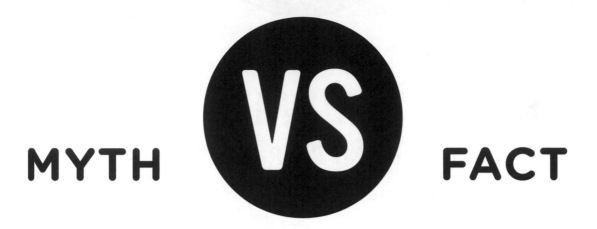

MYTH VS FACT

MYTH	FACT
In middle age, the best exercise regimen is lots of low- to moderate-intensity cardio and a little bit of lifting.	After age forty, strength training becomes more important than ever, for preserving muscle mass, avoiding injuries, and alleviating joint pain.
A person can gain sufficient muscle with cardio, such as walking on an incline or using the stair-stepper at the gym, because it uses bodyweight.	To build or maintain muscle mass in the upper and lower body, you need total-body strength training. Bodyweight circuits are good for this; and dumbbell and barbell workouts are best.
The older you get, the more exercise you must do to prevent weight gain and middle age spread.	With a more effective workout, you don't need to increase your exercise time. (But strength training should become an increasingly larger proportion of your exercise time as you age.)
Weight lifting is for bodybuilders—at my age, I'm likely to get hurt.	Significantly more injuries, especially overuse injuries, are reported from running rather than weight lifting each year.

You started losing muscle, naturally, after a certain age. For most people, muscle atrophy kicks in around forty-five. By the late fifties, men are losing an average of 4.2 pounds (1.9 kg) of skeletal muscle per decade. For women, it's less—around 2.4 pounds (1.1 kg)—but you probably had less muscle than men to begin with.[230]

Rather than working to preserve your muscle mass through strength exercises, you chose cardio—most people do—but it's the very type of exercise that does little, if anything, to increase muscle mass.[231-232]

Then you started dieting. Calorie restriction often *compounds* muscle loss.[233] So your resting metabolism probably began to dip.

Fully 80 percent of men and 75 percent of women ages thirty-five to seventy-four were at an unhealthy weight (BMI) at the last U.S. census.[234]

And what's the final nail in the coffin? It's doing the same cardio regimen for years. Your body adapted because you never progressed or varied your routine, so your metabolism basically decided to lie down and take a nap.

As you traded muscle for fat, your strength and vitality waned. With less power to push through your workouts, your once vigorous cardio routine became sluggish—and your energy expenditure did, too. (In fact, you probably hit the energy expenditure ceiling described in chapter 4 [see page 72].)

This is the recipe for getting fat in middle age. If you're here, at least you have company: fully 80 percent of men and 75 percent of women ages thirty-five to seventy-four were at an unhealthy weight (BMI) at the last U.S. census.[234]

But all hope isn't lost. Here's a pair of dumbbells.

THE RACE AGAINST THE CLOCK

As we enter our forties, we're not only concerned with being attractive; now we're also trying to stave off fat gain and heart disease. This leads many adults to pull back on strengthening exercise (if they even did it in the first place) and focus solely on cardio, believing this is what they need to shrink their bellies and protect their tickers. This scenario is all too common, and my heart breaks just thinking about it.

Middle age is exactly the time when men and women should be ramping up their strength training, not stopping. It's also the time when you have my permission to throw in the towel on cardio altogether!

The main reason is age-related muscle atrophy, as mentioned previously. Skeletal muscle is critical for preventing injuries and reducing risk of chronic diseases. It also plays a huge role in metabolism. So you can imagine that saying goodbye to muscle is not a good thing.

Over time, your metabolism will start to slow and it will become harder and harder for your body to burn fat. Maybe it has already.

Dwindling muscle then opens the door to injury. Workplace and household injuries are a concern for aging populations[235], and injuries, as we've seen, are the *norm* for runners and joggers.[236] This can spell the end of a well-meaning physical activity regimen.

Strength training has long been treated as a supplement to a workout routine, but, in fact, by itself delivers most of the benefits we seek from exercise:

- Protective boost against cardiovascular disease and metabolic syndrome

- Improved metabolism

- Strength and balance

- Confidence, energy, and attractiveness

- Psychological well-being

- Enhanced aerobic capacity

Are you surprised to see some of those on the list? Weightlifting and bodyweight exercises have been some of the best-kept secrets of the fitness world for too long. You might be shocked to find out how many of your favorite celebrities and models strength train to get their physiques (even Marilyn Monroe lifted weights). But increasingly, people are catching on. Let's look to the research to see why.

A NOTE ABOUT BONE DENSITY

If you want to stay strong and avoid injury at *any* age, bone density is your friend. Cardio exercise can help improve bone density, but usually only in the legs and, to a lesser extent, the spine. Just as exercisers who are completely focused on cardio tend to have weaker upper-body muscles, they can also suffer from weaker bone density in the arms and wrists, making them more susceptible to injury. Total body resistance exercise is critical for strengthening those vulnerable areas.

FAT LOSS AFTER FORTY *IS* POSSIBLE

We've been bombarded by so many claims from health experts about how we "need" cardio to lose weight that blunt refutes sometimes come as a shock.

Take one from Dr. Robert Lustig, who wrote in the bestselling book *Fat Chance* that there is more to weight loss than simply burning more calories.[237] He argues this is why banking on exercise-induced energy expenditure won't make people slim.

He's right. But what he didn't explain is that it isn't "cardio or bust."

Lustig painted a bleak picture of exercise altogether. But obviously, people can and *do* lose weight with certain forms of exercise.

We've seen the evidence on nearly every single page of this book.

True, exercise alone won't have everyone slipping back into the jeans they wore at age twenty. Body composition is a complex outcome with many predictors, including genes and chronic health conditions. Solving the puzzle gets even trickier as we age.

It is also true that our eating habits can complicate the results we get from exercise.[238] (Especially if said exercise leads you to mindlessly increase your calorie intake.) But that's fixable with an eating plan that complements your workout routine, which is where chapter 9 comes in.

We know that energy expenditure—or calories out—is not the only way that exercise helps the body shed excess fat. We expend energy at rest, but watching TV isn't making people fitter. Neither is walking for miles and miles a day, as Dr. Pontzer's studies pointed out (see chapter 4). But that's a strike against cardio, not exercise.

Obviously, Catherine isn't the only person to achieve a slimmer, fitter figure after forty through exercise and moderate changes to her diet. And her workout routine, as you've seen, is a mix of HIIT and strength training, just like the ones in this book.

Here's another glitch in the anti-exercise argument. Lustig wrote: "A second reason that exercise doesn't cause weight loss is that when you exercise, you build muscle. That's good for your health, but it doesn't reduce your weight."[239]

So you replaced fat with muscle mass and improved the contours of your body . . . what's the problem? Gaining muscle and losing fat at the same time is guaranteed to help you look more attractive. That's why it behooves us to talk about fat loss instead of "weight" loss.

Literally several dozens of studies show that even when weight loss is comparable between aerobic and strength-training programs, only strength training preserves or increases muscle.[240-241] And the fact is, even if you only gain muscle—with no fat loss whatsoever—you're in a much better place. (Though I'll be shocked if, barring other glaring factors, you were to follow the advice in this book and not lose fat. I haven't seen it.)

Gaining muscle and losing fat at the same time is guaranteed to help you look more attractive. That's why it behooves us to talk about fat loss instead of "weight" loss.

Yet over time—usually beyond the eight or twelve weeks of most exercise studies—you will likely see the numbers on the scale drop, too. For one, muscle increases your resting metabolism, so it helps your body burn fat. Those who are obese are even more likely to lose fat with increasing resistance exercise.[242]

Along the same lines, building muscle can help prevent fat gain in the future. Muscle loss is considered the biggest culprit behind

DOES WEIGHTLIFTING WORK FOR FAT LOSS?

There's plenty of debate about whether strength training really helps people lose fat. Some studies show it doesn't, but some show very convincing evidence that it does.

Older men who participated in a progressive strength-training program for sixteen weeks reduced both visceral and subcutaneous abdominal fat significantly—by 10.3 percent.[245] These men, all with type 2 diabetes, also had improved insulin sensitivity and lowered fasting blood glucose from their twice-a-week resistance workouts. And they got stronger.

Resistance training also helped premenopausal women maintain muscle after diet-induced weight loss.[246] Meanwhile, both the aerobic group and the control (no exercise) group lost muscle, strength, and even resting energy expenditure. This is why weight cycling (losing weight, only to gain it back) is so common among dieters who don't pair it with the right kind of exercise regimen. Long term, less muscle means your body will have a harder time keeping the weight off.

Purdue University similarly found that subjects age sixty and over could lose fat with resistance training.[247] Thirty-six men and women performed strength training three times a week for twelve weeks, doing exercises such as leg presses, chest presses, and seated rows: three sets, eight to twelve repetitions per set. At the same time, they consumed a 2,000-calorie diet.

Bodyweight stayed about the same, but participants lost four pounds (1.8 kg) of fat and gained four pounds (1.8 kg) of muscle. Yes, you can lose fat and gain muscle at the same time, at any age! Not only did increased muscle mass speed their fat loss, the strength-training regimen also improved blood sugar control by 25 percent, offering protection against diabetes.

a slowing metabolism as we age. Wayne Westcott, Ph.D., writes, "Inactive adults experience a 3 percent to 8 percent loss of muscle mass per decade, accompanied by resting metabolic rate reduction and fat accumulation."[243]

All of this is leading us to an important distinction: The focus of exercise shouldn't be pounds or inches. It should be body composition.

As Dr. Lustig acknowledged, what we care about at the end of the day are the changes in the body that the weight and inches can signify: improvements to our metabolic profile and reduced risk of chronic diseases.

But Lustig suggested that when studies show a decrease in body fat percentage from exercise, it might be because the proportion simply changes: If you add muscle mass, then fat will comprise a smaller *percent* of your body weight even if you don't lose fat.[244] However, most of the studies we've covered in this book reported not only increased muscle, but also fat loss (not weight loss). Scientists often measure loss of fat pounds with sophisticated tools in a lab setting, and they also use calipers to measure inches and "fat rolls" lost.

While HIIT is usually the most effective exercise for fat loss, as explained in chapters 2 and 4, strength training definitely adds fat-blasting power to your regimen. It helps you build or maintain muscle mass, keeping your metabolism going strong. Strength training can also raise your resting metabolic rate for several hours after your workout. (Recall the "afterburn" effect from chapter 4.)

LET'S TALK ABOUT SKINNY FAT

When John F. Kennedy said we needed to "move steadily toward a stronger and more vigorous America," he probably didn't have an army of scrawny elliptical riders in mind.[248]

Some people are thin because of muscle loss—due to inactivity, old age, or even excessive cardio. They might think they're in the clear. But while "skinny fat" people don't always get flagged as having a problematic body mass index, they're not much better off than their overweight counterparts. Thin doesn't automatically equal healthy.

A few years back, a reality TV show called *Fit to Live* put average Americans to the test. While many were overweight, the contestants also included people who fell in the "skinny

fat" camp. In simulations of real-life catastrophes, they fared just as poorly. They were so weak they couldn't save their own lives.

This is why the narrow view of exercise as a tool only to achieve weight loss and heart health is seriously problematic. Humans need muscle to promote bone and joint health. If you're strong, you'll have a lower risk of debilitating injuries. You might even face a real life-or-death situation. Will you be able to save yourself or your loved ones?

If you're an avid cyclist or runner and want to continue with your endurance sport, take heed. Adding strength training is a must to prevent muscle loss, which, as we've seen, can be compounded from a high volume of cardio.

And, if you're dieting, resistance training is critical to help preserve muscle during calorie restriction.[249] But there's no need to go on a diet, really: An efficient short burst workout routine and sensible approach to nutrition, like what I present in this book, should get you to your goals faster.

If you're an avid cyclist or runner and want to continue with your endurance sport, take heed. Adding strength training is a must to prevent muscle loss, which, as we've seen, can be compounded from a high volume of cardio.

IT'S NEVER TOO LATE TO BUILD MUSCLE

The good news is that it doesn't necessarily get harder to build muscle as you age. Jack LaLanne blew that myth out of the water when he pulled a 2,500-pound (1,134 kg) cabin cruiser *through* the water, for more than a mile, at age forty-three. In fact, LaLanne didn't start breaking fitness records until he was in his forties.

So did Catherine. She started doing my metabolic resistance training workouts in her mid-forties, and that was a few years ago. She's not only still doing them, she's teaching them to her clients, too!

It's never too late. Really.

Researchers at the University of Oklahoma put this to the test.[250] They found that men ages thirty-five to fifty significantly gained strength and muscle mass, right alongside the young eighteen to twenty-two year old men, in an eight-week strength-training program. Both groups increased their one-rep max and boosted muscle mass in the split upper-body and lower-body program. What's more . . . the middle-aged guys lost significantly more fat and decreased their body fat percentage more than the young guys!

We're always battling human nature. That's one reason people avoid resistance training in the first place. Or they choose puny weights (that barely weigh more than an office stapler), pump them in the air a few times, and think that's enough to build muscle. It's not.

The secret to an effective strength-training regimen is (surprise, surprise) intensity. The old idea that you need to wait forever between sets is false. Nor do you need to move slowly through your reps. Doing strength training in an interval fashion, with short burst movements, will get great results too.

Part of the equation is pushing yourself: lifting heavier weights or lifting lighter weights to fatigue. Strength and muscle gains come from steadily increasing your strength and ability to do more.

The current public health guidelines for strength exercise don't tell you this. In fact, they're so vague they make it simple to choose the easy route. There is no mention of intensity or duration. Thus, many people lift light weights and do exercises like sit-ups and crunches, rather than doing more efficient exercises that use your bodyweight and work multiple muscle groups at once.

Early proponents of aerobics were happy to let us get away with a few five-pound (2.3 kg) dumbbell curls and a sit-up here and there. Anything more intense than that, they suggested, was unnecessary—possibly even dangerous. Sorry, but you're not going to build much muscle from a regimen of cardio plus "light calisthenics." Just look at the lank physiques of older people who have been runners their whole lives.

In Spain, researchers observed significant strength gains in older men with type 2 diabetes who were following a resistance-training regimen.[251] They also reduced their abdominal fat and improved their insulin sensitivity after sixteen weeks. The same effects have been observed in older men without diabetes, too.[252] But the workout protocol in these studies followed the intensity principle: Twice a week, they did heavy resistance and "explosive" strength training and it was progressive. The point is, these men could do it in their sixties.

While it might not get harder to gain muscle from a *physiological* standpoint, I get it: You might feel weird at the gym. Maybe you're out of shape, or your gym clothes are out of style. Using the rowing machine in your "man cave" or the treadmill in the TV room is more appealing. But home workouts are great for strength training, as well. You can get away with as little as a few sets of weights, or just stick with bodyweight workouts.

BUSTING THE "WEIGHT LIFTING IS DANGEROUS" MYTH

And here's where I always get stopped. *But Craig*, people say. *Is weight lifting even safe at my age?*

Sigh.

You should really be asking, "Is it safe NOT to strength train at my age?"

The aerobics movement planted a fear of rigorous strength training in the hearts of Americans. That's one of the major reasons people eschew lifting in their forties, fifties, and sixties: Cardio is supposedly safer.

But the "danger" of weight lifting wasn't based on scientific evidence. In fact, there was barely any research to go from. The glorified claims about aerobic exercise led to few studies of anything else!

Thus, we can only guess that the negativity toward weight lifting was based on personal preference. What if influential figures, such as Dr. Kenneth Cooper, the "father of the modern fitness movement," simply didn't *like* it? (And in his seminal book, he says he didn't.) Thankfully, we now have plenty of research comparing different types of exercise that we can draw conclusions from.

Cardio pushers have long looked for evidence that people who lift weights are unhealthy. Dr. Cooper once mocked a bodybuilder for not being able to run a twelve-minute mile.[253] But, as Dr. Solomon and others have pointed out, the treadmill test was only ever an indicator of *aerobic* fitness, not a measure of health or any other kind of physical fitness capability.

Is weight lifting even safe at my age? *Sigh. You should really be asking, "Is it safe NOT to strength train at my age?"*

It's funny that the original argument against resistance training—that it wasn't good for anything other than resistance training—actually turned out to be true of aerobics!

Thankfully, Dr. Cooper came around: He started weightlifting at age fifty-five and still does today, in his eighties. "If you're going to be totally fit, you have to add weight training," he says.[254]

Now Cooper also instructs that, with each decade of age, people should devote a greater share of their workouts to strength training. It's the only way to keep your muscles and bones in good shape, according to the Cooper Institute's website, which currently offers ample strength training guidance.

There is one caveat. It's when people in their fifties who have been inactive for a while start exercising out of the blue that cardiac risk comes in. Too much exertion, too quickly, is considered a heart attack trigger, be it through running, shoveling snow, or even too much sexual activity when you're out of shape.[255] As has often been said, one of the best ways to prevent death by exercise . . . is to exercise.[256] But if you haven't been keeping up with it, then starting at a basic level and progressing properly is vital.

RESISTANCE EXERCISE *PREVENTS* INJURY

Not only is resistance exercise *not* dangerous when done properly, but it can help reduce injury and pain as you age—yet another reason to trade cardio for strength training after you make it "over the hill."

Strengthening your back and abdominals can help lessen back pain, as well as prevent work-related pain and strain and injuries due to strenuous activities encountered in everyday life.[257] Resistance training will also improve your balance, making you less prone to tumbles now and in old age.

Muscle helps protect the joints. Strengthening the leg muscles, for example, can prevent or alleviate arthritis in the knees. "Those muscles act as shock absorbers," writes Dr. Michael F. Roizen, of the Wellness Institute of the Cleveland Clinic.[258] "More muscle means fewer injuries, so you are more likely to stick to your routine and stay healthy."

If you have joint pain from years of running, strengthening the muscles in your legs can help alleviate the pain. We lose the most muscle from the lower body, as opposed to the upper body, as we age, making this especially important.[259] (Unless you want to keep the physical therapists, chiropractors, and orthopedic surgeons in business.)

The poor guy from chapter 5 who had to resign himself to an exercise bike in old age because his knees were busted up from years of running would've been better off stopping cardio altogether, and, instead, implementing a strength-training program.

WHY WOMEN AND WEIGHTS DO MIX

Tragically, even fewer women than men do strength training. In fact, and I almost can't believe this, many women are still being told *not* to do it.

RESISTING RESISTANCE TRAINING: A TROUBLING PICTURE

Only one-fourth of Americans are doing sufficient resistance exercise.[261] Sufficient, according to the U.S. government, means two strength exercise sessions per week—at any intensity, for any duration. As far as I can tell, pushing a loaded grocery cart through Costco would qualify as meeting the guideline.

Meanwhile, 50 percent are meeting the much more specific aerobic exercise guideline (150 minutes of moderate cardio or seventy-five minutes of vigorous cardio). They believe that cardio is more important. My bet is the same holds true for other countries.

The number of people doing the bare minimum of resistance exercise decreases with each generation. The proportion drops from 28 percent of eighteen to forty-four year olds doing some kind of strength exercise, to just 21 percent for those in the forty-five to sixty-four range. For those sixty-five and older, it hovers below 17 percent.

It's a disaster because resistance exercise is pretty much our only hope of staying strong, preventing frailty, and holding on to enough muscle to help stave off disease and fight fat—especially the dangerous, rock-hard belly fat that begins to set in after age forty.[262]

Even fewer women than men are meeting the strength training guideline—across every age group. There is one curious trend: Despite fairly large drops from younger generations to older ones, the number of women reporting regular resistance exercise stays constant between the fifty-six to sixty-four group and the sixty-five to seventy-four group. It even rises slightly for women after sixty-four. Maybe women who are living longer have strength training partly to thank?

There's a prevalent myth that women will bulk up from resistance exercise and should instead do light toning and cardio to "elongate" their muscles.

First things first, if your goal is fat loss, then ladies should know that you're even *less* likely to lose fat with cardio than men.[260] That's one reason that strength training, combined with HIIT, is a must.

Second, women don't bulk up with moderate resistance training, as I'll explain in the workout section. Instead, you build muscle that gives contours to your body. (Just Google your favorite female celebrity + "weight training" and you'll get proof!)

You'll also gain strength, the kind that will let you play with your kids and grandkids, travel the world, or avoid injury that could land you in a nursing home.

Once you're in your forties (or in your fifties, if you have exceptional genes), the repercussions of listening to these untruths start to wreak havoc.

STRENGTH TRAINING AND DISEASE PREVENTION

As you saw in chapter 2, reduction of excess body fat can go a long way in helping the body ward off disease. One of the scariest things to happen to our body in our forties and fifties, if we're not careful, is the formation of a hard, round belly. That gut isn't so harmless: Deep abdominal fat that lies below the muscle is associated with increased risk of heart and metabolic diseases.

Beyond shrinking toxic belly fat, physical activity is linked to improved health *independent* of fat loss, including lowered risk of diabetes, coronary heart disease, breast cancer, and colon cancer. Resistance training can help us claim all of these exercise benefits, and it also delivers a few extras, such as prevention of osteoporosis and arthritis.

Strength training also plays a role in cardiovascular health. It has been found to reduce systolic blood pressure in metabolic syndrome, according to a recent meta-analysis.[263] Of course, we might have guessed it by looking back to the seminal 1975 study of longshoremen, who were dying from significantly fewer cardiac events than their coworkers back in the office thanks to all that heavy lifting at the docks every day.[264]

Eight weeks of resistance exercise has been found to improve glucose control and fat oxidation, and to reduce liver fat, helping to reduce risk of cirrhosis.[265]

BOOST YOUR AEROBIC CAPACITY WITH KETTLEBELLS

Certain types of resistance training are also an efficient way to increase aerobic capacity. Kettlebell workouts are a great example, given the "explosive" nature of certain exercises.

For the uninitiated, a kettlebell is like a weighted cannonball with a handle. It's a versatile type of weight that makes it possible to do movements such as swings, lunges, and snatches, moving through a full-body range of motion—meaning they incorporate your whole body.

A study conducted by researchers at University of Wisconsin–La Crosse found that an eight-week kettlebell program improved aerobic capacity in a group of college-age male and female volunteers.[271] The study was sponsored by the American Council on Exercise, or ACE, which is a nonprofit that sponsors university-based exercise science research.

Participants did thirty to forty-five minutes of kettlebell exercises twice a week in a progressive format. That means they started with an amount of weight they could comfortably manage and advanced to a heavier weight when they were ready. The kettlebell group got a boost in aerobic capacity significantly different from the control group.

DISEASE RISK 101

Physical activity has been shown to reduce risk factors associated with chronic diseases, especially when exercise habits are regular and sustained in middle age and beyond. Some health concerns mitigated by exercise include the following:

Metabolic syndrome: Factors that increase risk of diabetes, coronary heart disease, and stroke, including:[266]

- Abdominal obesity
- High blood pressure
- Low HDL levels (beneficial cholesterol)
- High triglyceride levels (fat type in the blood)
- High fasting blood sugar
- Insulin resistance

Diabetes: This disease is caused by too much glucose in the blood; in diabetics, glucose that enters the blood from food *stays* there. The body doesn't produce insulin (type 1) or is unable to use it well (decreased insulin sensitivity, type 2) to regulate blood glucose (sugar). Regular exercise several times a week—including strength training—improves insulin sensitivity and has glucose-lowering effects.[267] Strength training can reduce visceral and subcutaneous abdominal fat significantly, which has been shown to improve insulin sensitivity and lower fasting blood glucose.[268]

Cancer: Reduced cancer risk from exercise may come from a combination of beneficial effects on obesity, insulin resistance, inflammation, and sex hormones. Highly physically active people have a 30 to 40 percent lower risk of developing colon cancer than sedentary individuals.[269] Physically active women have a 25 percent lower risk of breast cancer, on average, and higher-intensity exercise that promotes fat loss has the biggest impact on reducing breast cancer risk.[270]

John Porcari, Ph.D., who oversaw the study, said the improvement from kettlebells was better than walking, slightly less than running, and about on par with a cycling program.

Of course, that study used subjects in their early twenties. But University of Wisconsin–La Crosse teamed up with ACE for another study to test kettlebell workouts on men and women in their thirties and forties.[272] This time, participants did twenty minutes of continuous kettlebell exercise performed in interval-training fashion. Again, kettlebell workouts boosted aerobic capacity.

Participants achieved exercise heart rates that ranged from 86 to 99 percent of maximum heart rate and 67 to 91 percent of maximum oxygen uptake, meaning that kettlebells gave them a much higher-intensity workout than basic weightlifting.

Another study, this one published in *The Journal of Strength & Conditioning Research*, again found a boost to the cardiorespiratory system with kettlebell workouts, beyond what you'd get with circuit training.[273] But a boost in your maximal oxygen intake—which is one measure of cardiorespiratory performance—is merely a bonus of kettlebell exercises and similar dynamic, full-body resistance workouts. The real benefit is they're a very time-efficient and effective way to build muscle, compared with traditional weight lifting that often works single muscle groups in isolation (such as a biceps curl).

Kettlebell exercises are an especially great way to strengthen the abdominal muscles, or core.[274] The eight-week kettlebell regimen just referenced led to significant boosts in abdominal core strength in participants, as well as improved leg and grip strength, and even better balance. No wonder kettlebell workouts, which were invented by Russian strongmen in the 1800s, are making a comeback.

Kettlebell and bodyweight workouts are a particularly beneficial way to train for the over-forty crowd, given that improved core strength can help prevent or reduce lower back pain that kicks in as we age. They're also so efficient that they fit more easily into increasingly busy schedules.

OLDER BUT WISER

When Catherine first decided to try a short burst workout program, she didn't think she would enjoy it. In fact, she was skeptical that she could even do it at her age. The guide she had purchased stayed tucked inside a desk drawer right next to the treadmill for months.

After the "senior discount" moment at the grocery store, Catherine, in her forties, decided it was finally time to fold up the treadmill and try the HIIT program. Twelve weeks later, she had fitness results like she'd never seen, and she set another twelve-week goal from there.

Here's what Catherine said:

In just a few months, I've gone from middle-aged invisibility to ... hmm, I don't know what to call it because it's not the same as the attention that you get in your twenties that often makes you uncomfortable. It's more like being comfortable in your own skin, embracing who you are. Yes, that's it. The idea that after forty a woman should gracefully disappear from the spotlight is just stupid.

In the end, Catherine ended up being featured in an *ABC News* segment about extraordinary physical transformations. That's right: She achieved an "extraordinary transformation" by simply trading long cardio sessions for a more efficient HIIT and strength-training regimen—specifically, short burst workouts, such as the ones in this book, three times a week.

Some health experts have come to the sorry conclusion that exercise volume must increase, *indefinitely*, to compensate for age-related weight gain.[275] So you're up to one hour a day at age forty . . . two hours at fifty . . . and three hours by age sixty? Guess you'd better take an early retirement so you have time to do all that exercise!

And logging more and more miles on the treadmill might even have you looking the part—just like Catherine, who, remember, at the height of her cardio regimen was mistaken for a senior citizen at the grocery store . . . at age forty-four!

It's time to look past the cardio prescription. You *can* lose fat and gain muscle in your forties, fifties, sixties, and beyond . . . and you don't need to sacrifice sixty minutes of your life every day to do it.

With an efficient strength- and interval-training regimen, you can be in great shape well into your golden years.

WHAT YOU NEED TO KNOW

- Muscle helps the body prevent diseases, slows the accumulation of unhealthy body fat, and lessens the risk of injury and frailty.

- Muscle mass naturally begins to deplete in the mid-forties; the more you have stocked up, the better off you'll be.

- The traditional emphasis on cardio and little to no strength training is a recipe for flabby, overweight, unhealthy aging bodies—which is what we now have across America and most other places where people have adopted a Western lifestyle.

- The exercise trend is shifting, though. Strength training with weights ranked fourth among the ten top fitness trends of 2016, according to the American College of Sports Medicine . . . right behind wearable tech, HIIT, and bodyweight training.[276]

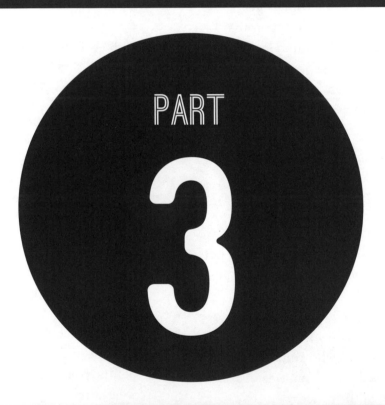

PART

3

A BETTER WAY

Your interval workouts never need to be longer than 20 minutes, and most take under 10 minutes.

8

YOUR NEW HIGH-INTENSITY TRAINING PROGRAM

DESPITE MY BEST efforts to spread the word about short burst workouts, I get the same question on Facebook every day: "Hey Craig, what's the best cardio for fat loss?" It saddens me when I get this question because it shows people are still being fooled into thinking they need hour-long cardio workouts on a near daily basis to get in shape. Of course you don't.

You're now ready to ditch the cardio and use real workouts that will get you losing fat, building muscle, and becoming the fitter, healthier person you want to be—without wasting precious hours in a boring (and ineffective) cardio regimen. In the following pages, you'll find three workouts: Bodyweight, Interval Training, and Metabolic Resistance. Each exercise is designed to get you maximum results in minimal time without the need for expensive gym memberships or equipment. Plus, they're fun, offering variety and keeping you focused and challenged. Before we get moving, I'll explain why they are so effective.

SCIENTIFICALLY PROVEN SECRETS TO GET MAXIMUM RESULTS IN MINIMAL TIME

One of the ways short burst workouts differ from steady-state cardio is they eliminate the "more is better" mentality. You shift your mindset from quantity to quality, and that eliminates your risk of overuse injuries.

The power of intense training of any kind is that it is efficient. One round of interval training or resistance training gets you more than 50 percent of the total results of the workout. Doing three rounds is not three times better, although multiple sets do give you more results than just one.

Your workouts are short and sweet (and sweaty) because increased workout intensity (quality) brings about rapid changes in your body. Including rest periods, your interval workouts never need to be longer than twenty minutes and most often take under ten minutes.

The power of intense training of any kind is that it is efficient.

Each workout in this section can be done as a standalone exercise program. Train three times per week and you'll get fit and lose fat. For advanced fitness and body composition goals, do the metabolic resistance training workouts followed by the four-minute bodyweight exercise circuit.

AVOIDING PLATEAUS

Doing the same exercises over and over again often leads to a plateau and overuse injuries. Smart personal trainers have clients switch resistance training exercises every three to four weeks. This also helps avoid overuse injury.

With the dozens of exercises and wide repetition range to use (you can get benefits from five to fifteen reps), there is an endless number of workouts you can do to overload your muscles and provide continual improvements in strength and body composition changes. For example, you could simply reverse the order of the exercises in your circuit routine or use slight variations of the exercises, and your workout will be as good as new.

WARMING UP

There is absolutely no need for a lengthy warm-up. (That's another aerobics-era myth that you can happily say goodbye to!)

- For the four-minute bodyweight workouts, doing one round of the exercises for a few repetitions is an adequate warm-up.

- For the metabolic resistance training or "MRT" workouts, a bodyweight exercise warm-up of mountain climbers, prisoner squats, and push-ups should be done first, followed by one set of each MRT exercise using 50 percent of the weight you'll use in the real sets. For example, if you're going to do Goblet Squats (page 147) with twenty pounds (9 kg) in your workout, then do a warm-up set using ten pounds (4.5 kg).

BODYWEIGHT WORKOUTS

When I started writing for *Men's Health* magazine in 2000, most of the workouts I created included dumbbell and even barbell exercises. Those were a reflection of my favorite ways to train as a college student with plenty of time—and equipment—available.

But I soon started receiving emails from men and women all over the world, of all ages, who complained they had no time to go to a gym and no fancy equipment at home . . . but still wanted to get results. That led me to a deep dive into the world of unique bodyweight exercises, so all of my readers could increase their fitness and burn fat at home without any equipment at all.

Soon, I started creating unique bodyweight workouts for major health and fitness magazines, and they were a huge hit with millions of readers. The bodyweight circuits in this book will give you fantastic fitness results in much less than an hour. In fact, try four minutes!

In an experiment published in *Applied Physiology, Nutrition, and Metabolism,* Canadian researchers tested a high-intensity interval bodyweight routine against thirty minutes of steady-state cardio. Two groups of college-aged women did four workouts per week for four weeks.[277]

- **Group A** ran for thirty minutes at 85 percent max heart rate (hard cardio!).

- **Group B** did eight rounds of twenty seconds of a single bodyweight exercise (burpees, jumping jacks, mountain climbers, or squat thrusts) with ten seconds of rest between rounds.

The results? Both training groups increased their aerobic fitness levels by about the same amount (7 percent for endurance and 8 percent for bodyweight). That's right, the short bodyweight workouts (of four minutes) worked just as well for aerobic improvement as thirty minutes of cardio, even though they were seven times shorter.

But it was only Group B—those who did the bodyweight exercises—that also increased muscular endurance. And finally, this short burst style of training used by Group B also resulted in greater overall workout enjoyment compared to the cardio group and a greater intention to stick with it!

Scientists concluded that "extremely low-volume bodyweight interval-style training" will boost cardiovascular fitness just as well as slow, boring cardio while giving you better improvements in muscle endurance . . . all in just four minutes.

THE
WORKOUTS: BODYWEIGHT

Following are two of my favorite bodyweight workouts. They require no equipment, so you can literally do them anytime, anywhere, to get fit and lose fat. (I've even done them in airport lounge shower rooms in countries all over the world!) These total-body movements are designed to work many major muscle groups at once so you get more bang for your exercise buck than with aerobics. By doing the exercises in short bursts at high intensity, you'll also improve your cardio-vascular fitness and health.

Four-Minute Metabolic Miracle

Prisoner Squat—60 seconds

Spiderman Push-up or Kneeling Push-up—
    60 seconds

Total Body Extension—60 seconds

Cross-Body Mountain Climber—
    60 seconds

Four-Minute New-School Cardio and Abs

Total Body Extension—60 seconds

Rocking Plank—60 seconds

Run in Place or Jumping Jacks—
    60 seconds

Mountain Climber—60 seconds

HOW TO PERFORM EACH EXERCISE

Correct form is important to achieving results. Do not hold your breath while exercising. Inhale during the lowering phase and exhale on the exertion as you push back to the start position.

FOUR-MINUTE METABOLIC MIRACLE

PRISONER SQUAT

1. Stand with your feet slightly wider than shoulder-width apart.
2. Clasp your hands behind your head.
3. Keep your elbows back and shoulder blades pulled together to work the upper back.
4. Push your hips backward as if sitting into a chair.
5. Squat as deeply as possible, but do not let your lower back round.
6. Push through your heels and use the big muscles of your legs (your thighs and butt) to return to the starting position.

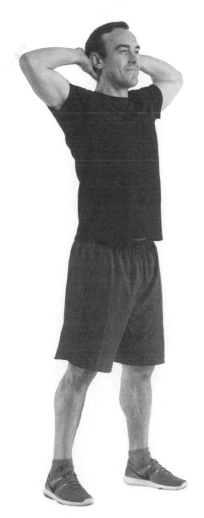
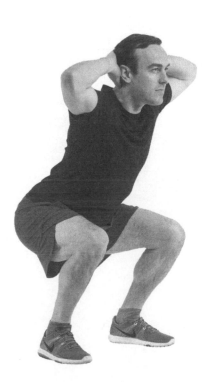

SPIDERMAN PUSH-UP

1. Place your hands on the floor slightly wider than shoulder-width apart.

2. Start at the top of a push-up position with your body in a straight line from toes to shoulders.

3. Brace your abs as if someone was about to punch you in the stomach, but breath normally. Slowly lower your body until you are one inch (2.5 cm) off the ground.

4. As you lower your body, slowly bring your right knee up to your right elbow, keeping your foot off the ground as you do so.

5. Push through your chest, shoulders, and triceps to return to the starting position and return your leg to the starting position.

6. Repeat, alternating sides.

7. Keep your body in a straight line at all times and do not twist your hips.

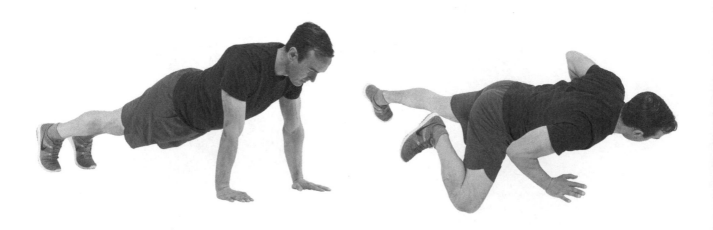

KNEELING PUSH-UP

1. Place your hands on the floor slightly wider than shoulder-width apart.

2. Keep your abs braced and your body in a straight line from toes to knees to shoulders. Keep your knees on the floor about hip-width apart.

3. Slowly lower your body until you are one inch (2.5 cm) off the ground.

4. Push through your chest, shoulders, and triceps to return to the starting position.

5. Keep your body in a straight line at all times.

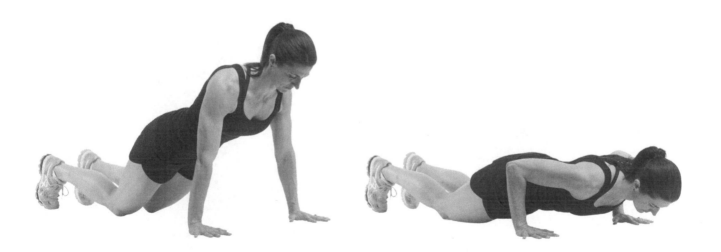

TOTAL BODY EXTENSION

This is a non-impact replacement for jumping.

1. Start in the standing position as if you were going to do a bodyweight squat.
2. Drop down quickly into a quarter squat and swing your arms behind you by your sides.
3. Explode up and extend your body onto your toes, raising your arms overhead.
4. Descend back into the quarter squat before exploding back up again.

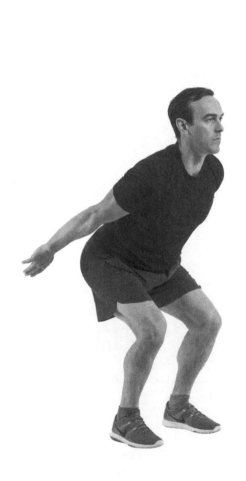
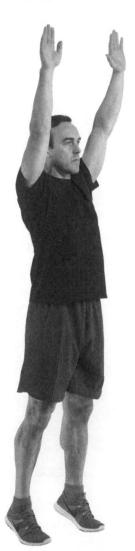

CROSS-BODY MOUNTAIN CLIMBER

1. Start at the top of the push-up position. Brace your abs.
2. Raise one foot off the floor and slowly bring your knee up to your opposite elbow.
3. Keep your abs braced and do not let your hips drop down.
4. Slowly return your leg to the starting position while keeping your abs braced.
5. Repeat, alternating sides.
6. If you get tired, drop down into a regular plank position.

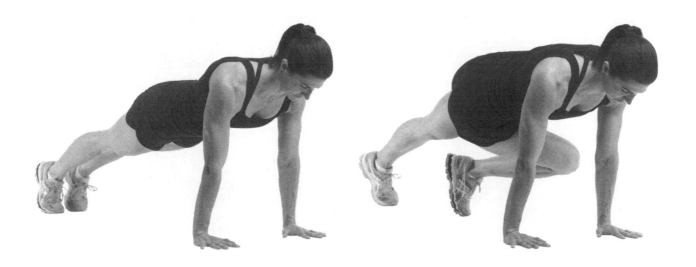

FOUR-MINUTE NEW-SCHOOL CARDIO AND ABS

TOTAL BODY EXTENSION

This is a non-impact replacement for jumping.

1. Start in the standing position as if you were going to do a bodyweight squat.
2. Drop down quickly into a quarter squat and swing your arms behind you by your sides.
3. Explode up and extend your body onto your toes, raising your arms overhead.
4. Descend back into the quarter squat before exploding back up again.

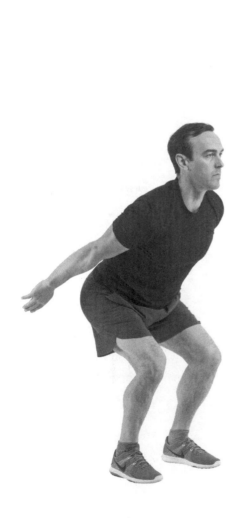
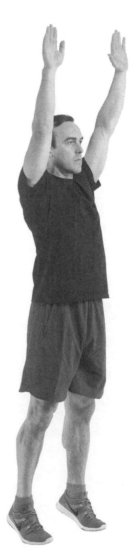

ROCKING PLANK

1. Support your bodyweight on your forearms and toes.
2. Brace your abs tightly so your body hovers over the mat.
3. Keep your back straight and your hips up.
4. Shift forward so your chest moves toward your hands.
5. Then shift back into the traditional plank position.
6. Repeat this rocking motion while keeping your abs braced.

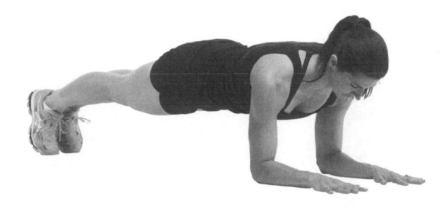

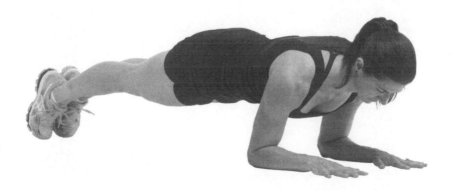

JUMPING JACKS

1. Start with your hands by your side and feet together.
2. Lift your arms over your head and jump your feet out to a wide-stance position.
3. Return arms and legs to the starting position.
4. Keep your chest up, abs braced, and stay light on your feet.

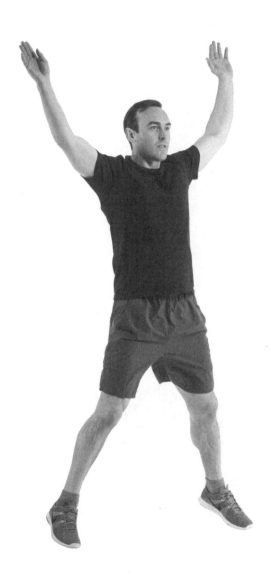
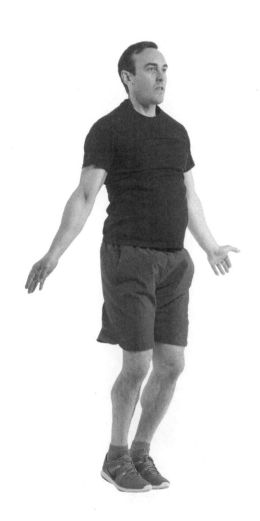

MOUNTAIN CLIMBER

1. Start at the top of the push-up position. Brace your abs.
2. Raise one foot off the floor and slowly bring your knee up to your chest.
3. Do not let your hips drop or rotate.
4. Keep your abs braced and slowly return your leg to the starting position.
5. Repeat, alternating sides.

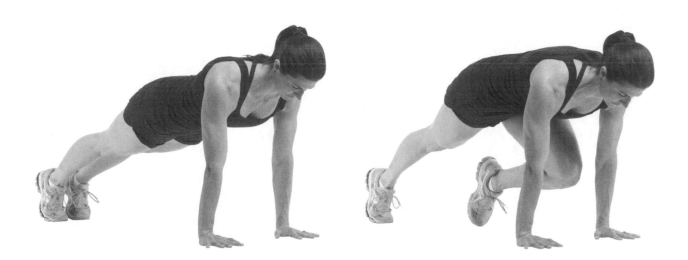

THE MYTH ABOUT WOMEN AND BULKING UP

Some women worry that strength training will make them look too muscular. I guarantee this won't happen with bodyweight training.

Female bodybuilders gain a lot of muscle because they eat more than truck drivers, lift more than 95 percent of guys at the gym do, and, quite possibly, take more steroids than Arnold ever used. In fact, the formula for getting big and bulky goes like this:

high volume of food $\times$ high volume of moderate- to high-intensity weight training ($\times$ extra male hormones) = muscle mass

Getting stronger doesn't mean getting bigger. Bruce Lee was very strong and powerful, but no one would call him a hulk. Female gymnasts are also strong and powerful, but without the bulk. Most women will never have too much muscle as a problem. If anything, bodyweight exercises and metabolic resistance training will help you get leaner and put curves in all the right spots.

Here's the unpopular truth: If a woman is gaining bulk, it's the weight on the fork that is the cause. Never forget that diet is more important than exercise for weight loss.

INTERVAL TRAINING WORKOUTS

The year was 1999, and it was the greatest year of my life. I was a graduate student in the exercise physiology department of McMaster University, with a side gig as the school's strength and conditioning coach. My job, if you could call it that, was to take the men's and women's basketball and soccer teams through their workouts.

In early April, with exams approaching and the summer season right after, my buddies on the soccer team needed to get fit fast. Fortunately, I had the answer.

I had just spent the last four months reading dozens of research papers about interval training. It had been around for decades, but hardly anyone was using it with athletes. Most coaches were stuck on the long, slow cardio approach to conditioning. But cardio doesn't lead to sport-specific fitness, it requires a lot of time, and it often leaves the athlete injured (and bored out of their young minds).

The solution was to take my friends and put them through thrice-weekly interval training workouts. We met on the soccer field after class, and just twenty minutes later we were done. They were whooped.

The workout included thirty to sixty seconds of interval runs followed with three times that duration spent in a walking recovery (using the "peaks and valleys" approach mentioned earlier). As they got fitter each session, we ran faster and rested less until we were down to a 1:1 work-to-rest ratio after just two to three weeks. They all felt like they were in mid-season form before the pre-season even ended.

Plus, because the conditioning was more sport-specific than the slow pace of boring cardio (and not done on a cardio machine), the athletes also got faster and were able to avoid injury that season.

But you don't need to exercise as much as these athletes if you want to lose fat and get fit. A 2016 study documented fat loss in an HIIT regimen of just four minutes of intense exertion a *week*. Not per session—per week. This proves how extremely efficient HIIT can be.[278] The subjects also lost fat without any restriction of food intake.

The benefits of HIIT workouts aren't limited to fat loss. In another 2016 study, this one led by Dr. Jenna Gillen and overseen by Dr. Martin Gibala, interval training delivered the same health gains as traditional endurance training.[279] Both groups gained the same amount of cardiorespiratory fitness and improved insulin sensitivity. This is incredible, given that the interval group did just one minute of intense exertion per workout. The short burst workout involved three twenty-second all-out cycle sprints, interspersed with two minutes of low intensity cycling, plus a few minutes of warming up and cooling down. The total time commitment was ten minutes, three days a week. The endurance exercisers did forty-five minutes of continuous cycling per workout, three days a week. Across the twelve-week training period, the endurance group logged twenty-seven hours of cycling, while the short burst group logged only thirty-six minutes of strenuous cycling *total*.

SO WHAT IS INTENSE EXERTION?

How do you know if your high-intensity intervals are high enough to burn fat? "High-intensity" is a subjective term. In other words, your high intensity is probably different from mine (see box, page 143).

I'll explain how to rate your workouts in a second; first, let's take a look at the research. Drs. Trapp and Boutcher and their Australian colleagues found that a tough yet tolerable version of an HIIT workout can deliver incredible fat-burning results.[280] Their subjects were predominantly sedentary women. They exercised hard for eight seconds and then recovered for twelve seconds. This cycle was repeated over and over for twenty minutes. They used special bikes, as this interval duration is difficult to program into an exercise bike you'll find at your local gym. However, it's instructional. You simply have to exercise hard for a short burst and alternate that with

GAUGING INTERVAL INTENSITY

Here's a simple protocol to gauge your intensity:

- Use the ten-point Borg Rating of Perceived Exertion Scale ("RPE Scale" for short) that ranges from zero to ten, where zero is loafing on the couch, five is moderate, and ten is exercising at an all-out pace.[282]

- When you do your intervals, you should be working at an eight or nine out of ten intensity. I explain to my clients that six out of ten is a regular cardio pace and ten out of ten is maximum exertion . . . but you don't need to train at that level because you could hurt yourself at that intensity (it's reserved for running for your life).

- Your goal for interval training is to exercise at a controlled, intense pace that is noticeably harder than normal cardio. Do this for one minute (if at an eight out of ten rating) or thirty seconds (if at a nine out of ten rating). Then drop the intensity of exercise down to a three out of ten for your recovery periods (a stroll in the park pace).

- Don't give in to the temptation to exercise hard during the recovery period, or you risk turning your interval training back into traditional cardio. Keep it very easy. Your workout should resemble peaks (intense effort) and valleys (easy recovery), not a steady level of intensity.

easy periods of exercise. The women in this study did their HIIT workout three times per week and after fifteen weeks, had significantly reduced total body fat, leg and trunk fat, and insulin resistance.

Dr. Gibala, whose studies have become so famous they have graced the pages of the *New York Times*, originally had his subjects do thirty-second nausea-inducing bouts of intervals interspersed with four minutes of recovery, but eventually discovered this level of sacrifice wasn't necessary for the average person just looking to get fit and have less fat. In follow-up studies, his subjects were able to

obtain similar results using one minute of tolerable intervals alternated with one minute of recovery.[281] This was still a far better approach than doing slow cardio.

A bonus benefit of interval training is that your workouts will fly by compared to a regular steady-state cardio session. The constant up-and-down nature keeps your mind occupied and, before you know it, your session will be over (plus, interval workouts are already shorter than cardio by at least half). Even better, you'll start seeing results—in both appearance and daily fitness, such as climbing stairs—in just days.

THE
WORKOUTS: INTERVAL TRAINING

An HIIT workout can be done with traditional cardio movements (like running, cycling, rowing, or swimming), kettlebell swings, or bodyweight circuits. Choose an exercise and intensity that causes fatigue in thirty to sixty seconds. This could be a hill sprint, a treadmill sprint, a stationary bike against resistance, bodyweight squats, or burpees—and these are just a few possibilities.

A three-minute warm-up and cool-down are all you need (whether you're doing cardio or not), and you're done in under twenty minutes.

The simplest cardio machine interval workout goes like this: six rounds of sixty-second work intervals (at an eight out of ten intensity), each followed by sixty-second recovery intervals (at a three out of ten intensity).

My favorite bodyweight interval workout is called "Punisher Squats." You'll do eight rounds of squats for twenty seconds, each followed by a ten-second "hold" in the bottom position. Your thighs have never experienced anything like this before!

A great kettlebell interval workout goes like this: thirty seconds of kettlebell swings followed by thirty seconds of active recovery (walk around in a circle at a slow pace). Repeat six times and you're done in six minutes flat.

KETTLEBELL SWING

1. Stand with your feet wider than shoulder-width apart.

2. Hold a single kettlebell (or dumbbell) in both hands in front of your body at arm's length.

3. Keep your abs braced and your lower back in a flat position at all times.

4. Push your hips back and "hike" the kettlebell between your legs.

5. Drive your hips back and keep a slight bend in your knees. The movement comes from the hips, not the knees, and is not a squat motion.

6. Drive your hips forward and stand back up to the starting position as you swing the kettlebell up to chest height. Move at a quick pace.

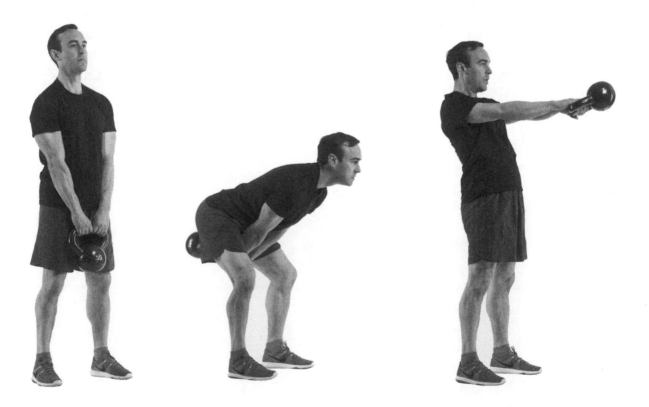

METABOLIC RESISTANCE TRAINING

Remember the first time you saw a simple magic trick? To the magician, it was nothing, but to the audience it was amazing and left them scratching their heads in awe. Well, metabolic resistance training is my magic trick.

You see, most clients come to me after spending years in a love–hate (mostly hate) relationship with cardio. But that doesn't work for weight loss. One reason it doesn't work is because regular cardio is done at a low intensity, and, therefore, it doesn't cause excess post-exercise energy consumption (known as EPOC, or afterburn, as described in chapter 4). The afterburn is the secret ingredient in my fat-burning metabolic workout magic trick.

When clients do their first metabolic resistance workouts under my watchful eye, they exercise at a higher intensity than they ever have before. As a result, they experience a greater build-up of metabolites (waste products from energy production) in their muscle and lactate in their blood (which may lead to nausea, so you have to be conservative and cutting-edge at the same time with these workouts). Metabolic resistance training also leads to a muscle pump (a neat feeling of increased blood accumulation in the muscles), in addition to the afterburn.

The afterburn has the greatest impact on fat loss. Clients often report a higher body temperature for hours after a metabolic workout . . . while this does not happen after cardio. It's like they can feel the accelerated fat burning going on for hours as they recover on the couch, watching television.

It's like magic.

But as a fitness magician, I know how it really works. It's not magic at all—just sweet, sweaty science.

So, what is metabolic resistance training, or MRT? MRT is a hybrid of traditional strength training and interval training. It can include bodyweight exercises, but usually refers to a circuit of dumbbell exercises (as in our sample workout).

The afterburn is the secret ingredient in my fat-burning metabolic workout magic trick.

Anytime you use supersets (pairs of exercises done without rest) or circuits (three exercises or more in a row without rest), you are doing metabolic resistance training. Similar to interval training, this causes metabolites to build up in the muscle cells. The muscle cells adapt by becoming better at producing energy, developing force (getting stronger), and clearing the metabolites. Over time, with repeated training, this makes you stronger and gives you more stamina.

THE
WORKOUTS: METABOLIC RESISTANCE

Workout 1

Goblet Squat—60 seconds

Cross-Body Mountain Climber—
   60 seconds

Dumbbell Row—30 seconds per side

Plank—60 seconds

Workout 2

Kettlebell Swing—60 seconds

Push-Up—60 seconds

Dumbbell Split Squat—30 seconds
   per side

One-Arm Standing Dumbbell Press—
   30 seconds per side

WORKOUT 1

GOBLET SQUAT

1. Stand with your feet slightly wider
   than shoulder-width apart.

2. Hold a dumbbell in a "cupped goblet"
   position at chest height.

3. Start the movement at the hip joint
   and push your hips backward as if
   sitting into a chair.

4. Squat as deeply as possible, but
   keep your lower back tensed in a neutral
   position. Don't let your lower back
   become rounded.

5. Push with your glutes, hamstrings,
   and quadriceps to return to the
   starting position.

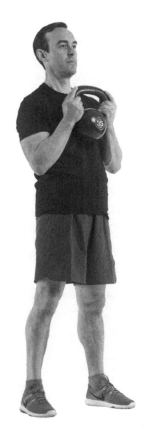
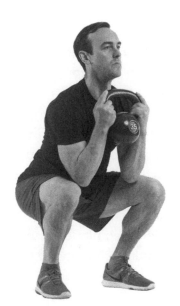

CROSS-BODY MOUNTAIN CLIMBER

1. Start at the top of the push-up position. Brace your abs.
2. Raise one foot off the floor and slowly bring your knee to your opposite elbow.
3. Keep your abs braced and do not let your hips drop down.
4. Slowly return your leg to the starting position while keeping your abs braced.
5. Repeat, alternating sides.
6. If you tire, drop down into a regular plank position.

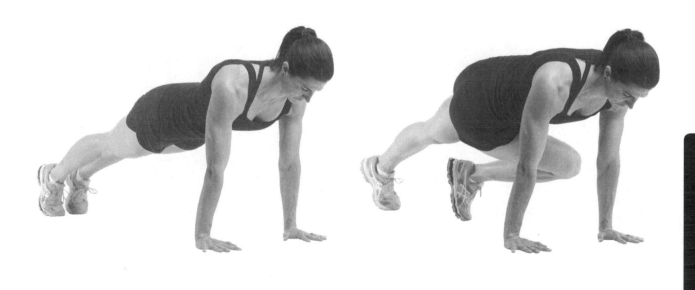

DUMBBELL ROW

1. Rest your left hand and left knee on a flat bench.
2. Lower your chest until it is parallel to the bench and keep your back flat.
3. Hold the dumbbell in the right hand at full extension and slowly row it up to the lower abdomen.
4. Keep your lower back tensed in a neutral position and keep your right elbow tight against your side.
5. Slowly lower and repeat.
6. Do not round your lower back.
7. Do thirty seconds for one side and then switch to the other side for thirty seconds.

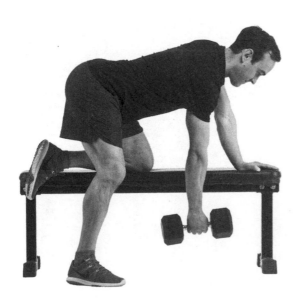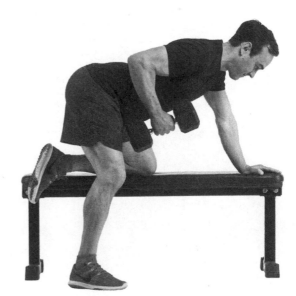

PLANK

1. Support your bodyweight on your forearms and toes.
2. Brace your abs tightly so your body hovers over the mat.
3. Keep your back straight and your hips up.
4. Hold this position for the recommended amount of time.

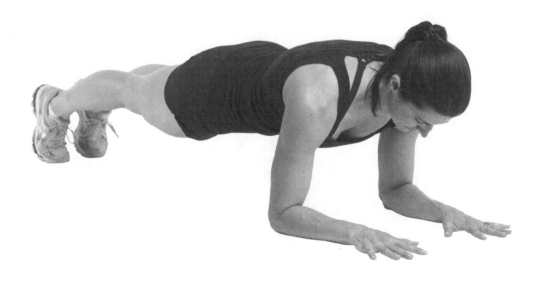

METABOLIC REISTANCE TRAINING

WORKOUT 2

KETTLEBELL SWING

1. Stand with your feet wider than shoulder-width apart.

2. Hold a single kettlebell (or dumbbell) in both hands in front of your body at arm's length.

3. Keep your abs braced and your lower back in a flat position at all times.

4. Push your hips back and "hike" the kettlebell between your legs.

5. Drive your hips back and keep a slight bend in your knees. The movement comes from the hips, not the knees, and is not a squat motion.

6. Drive your hips forward and stand back up to the starting position as you swing the kettlebell up to chest height. Move at a quick pace.

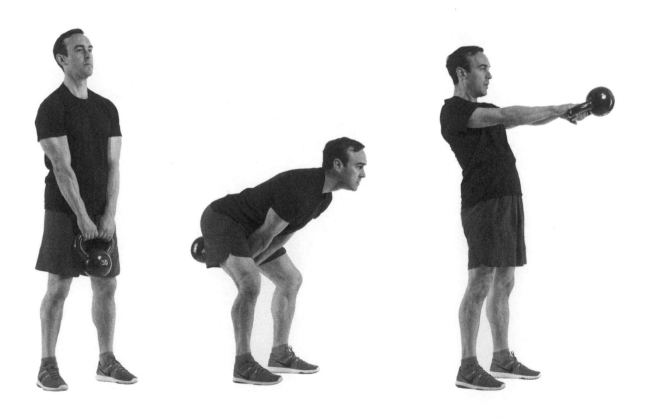

PUSH-UP

1. Place your hands on the floor slightly wider than shoulder-width apart.
2. Keep your abs braced and body in a straight line from toes to shoulders. Slowly lower your body until you are one inch (2.5 cm) off the ground.
3. Push through your chest, shoulders, and triceps to return to the starting position.
4. Keep your body in a straight line at all times.

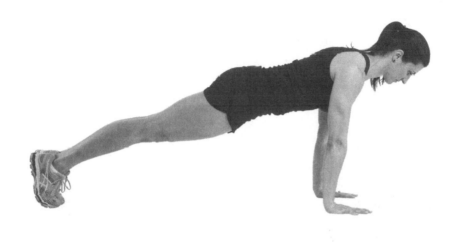

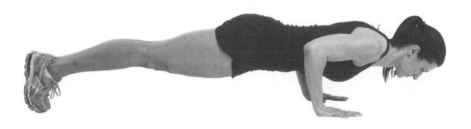

DUMBBELL SPLIT SQUAT

1. Stand with your feet shoulder-width apart and hold a dumbbell in each hand.
2. Step forward with your one leg, taking a slightly larger than normal step.
3. Press the ball of your back foot into the ground and use it to help keep your balance. The back knee should also be bent.
4. Brace your abs and keep your lower back flat (in a neutral position). Do not let it round forward.
5. Keep your upper body upright and lower your hips straight down until your front thigh is parallel to the ground.
6. Push through the heel of the front leg to return to the upright position, but don't step back. Stay in a split-squat stance.
7. Do thirty seconds for one side and then switch to the other side for thirty seconds.

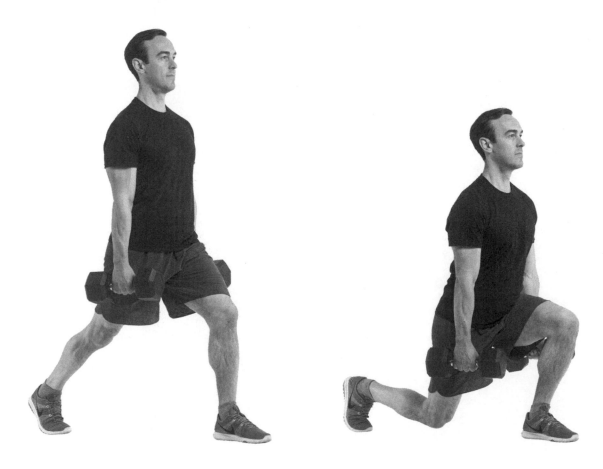

ONE-ARM STANDING DUMBBELL PRESS

1. Stand with your abs braced and knees slightly bent.
2. Hold one dumbbell at shoulder level with your palm turned toward your head.
3. Place the other hand on your abs as a cue to keep your abs braced.
4. Keep your elbow tucked against your body and press the dumbbell overhead.
5. Slowly lower to the starting position and repeat.
6. Do thirty seconds for one side and then switch to the other side for thirty seconds.

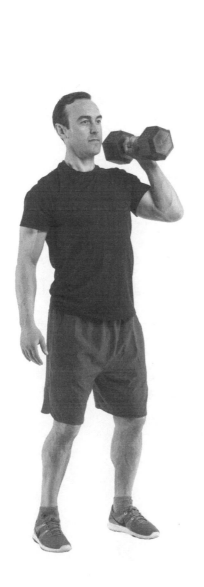
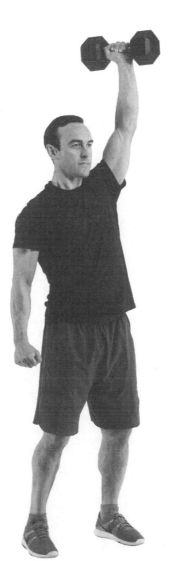

The typical fast food meal contains 1,200 to 3,000 calories.

9

WHAT YOU EAT MATTERS

A **S YOU LEARNED** in chapter 6, no amount of physical activity will save you if you're eating too many calories.

But this isn't the part where I tell you to go on a diet. Not at all. I don't advocate for starvation or restriction diets because they're often limiting, confusing, frustrating, or just plain annoying. Research actually backs me up on this.[283] One reason many popular diet programs fail is there are too many rules, plus a complete restriction of your favorite foods—which isn't necessary and is often detrimental.

I believe a nutrition plan should be simple, just like an exercise plan, because the key to success is following a set of principles you can stick with every day. That's why I recommend Chef Gui Alinat's *Eat More, Burn More* cookbook (you'll see an example on page 161). It shows you how to eat your favorite meals while still supporting weight loss.

The good news is that when you combine simple nutrition with short burst workouts, you can lose unwanted body fat quickly. In turn, this will boost your physical energy and mental alertness, making the quality of your workouts even better, further inspiring you to keep eating healthy foods.

So here are the New Rules of Dieting: No extreme calorie reductions and no cutting out food groups. And you can still enjoy some of your favorite indulgences. You don't need to go drastically "low fat" or "low carb." Whether you're gluten-free or not, dairy or no dairy, vegetarian or a fan of meat-eating Paleo diets, you can get healthy and lose belly fat with almost any sensible approach to eating. There is no "one best way" to eat for everyone, but there's often one best way that suits your schedule and preferences—while still getting results.

Whether you're gluten-free or not, dairy or no dairy, vegetarian or a fan of meat-eating Paleo diets, you can get healthy and lose belly fat with almost any sensible approach to eating.

Because there are many terrific nutrition guides out there, and I'm just a humble farm boy turned exercise scientist, I'll keep this short, sharing with you the main nutrition principles I use that will complement your exercise regimen and have you slim, strong, and healthy in no time.

AVOID THE AMERICAN DIET

I'm not the first person to recommend a sensible whole-foods diet, and I won't be the last, but it bears repeating. If you continue following the modern American approach to food—most meals prepared outside the home, tons of processed and man-made ingredients, and eating more calories than you need—then the workouts in this book will barely make a dent in your waistline. Sorry. Nutrition really is the most important factor in fat loss.

Let's look back at when I tried to "outrun pizza" in chapter 6. I burned forty calories running *as fast as I could*, while my friend Brad managed to eat 800 calories in the same amount of time—all in one slice of pizza and a large soda!

This is the downside of our busy lives. Americans increasingly eat food prepared away from home, and "away" food is loaded with more calories and more total and saturated fat than home-prepared meals.[284]

Here's something else that's alarming. Today, per-person cheese consumption in the United States is radically higher than it was three decades ago, and the United States Department of Agriculture (USDA) chalks it up to the increased popularity of commercially prepared foods, such as pizza, nachos, and fast-food sandwiches—which account for two-thirds of cheese use in America.[285] Hurray for Wisconsin! Boo for your belly.

And then there's fast food. Fast food is hands-down the biggest culprit of calorie

THINK ABOUT "DIET + EXERCISE"

Rather than think of it as "exercise versus diet," think about diet *plus* exercise because, as you saw in chapter 6, they go hand in hand.

Most important, you have to overcome the mentality of "I've burned it, so I've earned it." I've had clients who, in the past, would go immediately to Starbucks for Frappuccinos and biscotti after their workouts. We're talking upward of 500 calories . . . way more than they would have burned off even during one of my intense short burst workouts.

And forget about doing a Thanksgiving turkey trot or Black Friday marathon to burn off a 2,500-calorie holiday meal. Repeat after me: The "cardio confessional" never works.

But choosing exercise you enjoy should fix the need to reward yourself after your workouts. Counting how many cupcakes a sweat session "earned" seems to be a phenomenon unique to long, boring cardio! You might find that changing your exercise routine actually makes some of your nutrition choices easier. Often, carb cravings and appetite decrease, if you were doing tons of steady-state exercise before.

It's useful to keep an eye on how your workouts affect what you eat. It also pays to plan ahead and have your post-workout meal, whether breakfast, lunch, or a protein smoothie, prepared in advance so you can avoid grabbing unhealthy food in the name of convenience.

over-consumption in Western society.[286-287] A single fast-food meal contains 1,200 to 3,000 calories. Processed and packaged foods are filled with sugar and highly processed carbohydrates that contribute to deadly belly fat (a.k.a. visceral fat) and heart disease (and when you combine a marathoner's "good excuse" to eat high-carbohydrate processed foods for "recovery," you get a double whammy against your heart health and body fat).

But soda might be the worst culprit. In the 1990s, soft drink consumption skyrocketed more quickly than *any other food group*.[288] (Though pizza was a close contender, up 150 percent from the prior two decades.) Soda accounts for one-third of total added sugars consumed in America![289]

I guarantee if you trade these Western "staples" for a diet full of healthy, high-fiber, and low-sugar whole foods, you'll be in great shape.

What does that healthier diet look like? It's vegetables, fruit, nuts, and whole grains (unless you're gluten sensitive) as your foundation, complemented by high-quality protein sources, such as eggs, meat, and fish. If you eat bread, pastas, and oatmeal, skip the processed versions and choose high-fiber versions instead.

DO I NEED TO COUNT CALORIES?

It's a question people ask me all the time, and my answer is: It depends. Personally, I don't count calories. I haven't since I was a beginner following Arnold's bodybuilding bible back at the age of sixteen. For me, following simple nutrition rules and an exercise regimen that supports healthy eating have been enough to stay in great shape.

But I started out counting my calories. There's often great value in doing so, even just for a short time. Today, I can accurately eyeball the calorie counts in any given meal, even at the steakhouses I visit every other week for a special meal. Keeping track gives you a sense of what you're eating, so you can get back in touch with the nutrients and calorie amounts in different types of food. It also helps with planning, which is important for staying on track with your goals. You don't have to do it forever; a couple of weeks are enough.

Calorie tracking also gives you the chance to adjust if you're not seeing the results you want or if you hit a plateau. And as we saw in chapter 6, most people are eating way more calories than they realize.

Swapping the Western diet staples of fast food and processed food for fresh whole foods automatically cuts caloric intake by hundreds of calories a day. There's no math needed!

Another secret to success is food journaling. In a study from Kaiser Permanente of 1,700 participants, the people who kept a daily food diary lost twice as much weight as those who didn't.[290] Food journaling helps you see not only what you ate, but also *why* you ate it. Were you hungry? Bored? Stressed? Eating because your friends were eating?

Here's what prompted Catherine to start food journaling:

I am a compulsive overeater. One of my earliest memories is actually of a binge on white bread. I was climbing up on the kitchen counter and, literally, sneaking and stealing food as early as five or six years old. I can't really blame my parents for that. There was something biological about me that I could, literally, at age five, eat half a loaf of Wonder bread. I only stopped because I knew if I ate more I would get busted.

Knowing this, Catherine used a food journal to stay self-aware, and she says it was an important part of her transformation, helping her spot habits that were holding her back.

If you're not ready to think about counting calories or food journaling . . . just spend some time focusing on eating less low-quality food and more high-quality food. For many people, swapping the Western diet staples of fast food and processed food for fresh whole foods automatically cuts caloric intake by hundreds of calories a day. There's no math needed!

A TYPICAL DAY'S MEALS   *Courtesy of Chef Gui Alinat, author of* Eat More, Burn More

Here's proof that eating a sensible diet doesn't have to be miserable.

WOMEN: SAMPLE DAILY CALORIC REQUIREMENT: 1,800*

EXAMPLE 1 | TOTAL CALORIES: 1,780

Breakfast
Steel Cut Oatmeal & Fruit: 330 Calories

Lunch
Caprese Salad with Burrata: 370 Calories

Snack
2 Hardboiled Eggs: 160 Calories

Dinner
Braised Beef with Tomatoes & Olives: 610 Calories

Dessert
Greek Yogurt with Berries & ½ ounce (15 g) Walnuts:
310 Calories

EXAMPLE 2 | TOTAL CALORIES: 1,780

Breakfast
Baked Eggs with Salsa Verde: 250 Calories
Half an Avocado or 2 Small Pieces of Fruit:
170 Calories

Lunch
Grilled Corn & Summer Vegetable Salad: 400 Calories

Snack
1 ounce (30 g) Almonds & 1 Square Dark Chocolate:
260 Calories

Dinner
Green Bean Casserole: 220 Calories
Caramelized Brussels Sprouts: 170 Calories

Dessert
Apple with 2 tablespoons (32 g) Almond Butter:
310 Calories

Based on the average calorie requirement for women, which varies depending on metabolism, exercise level, and other factors. Use a free online app to calculate your daily calorie needs.

MEN: SAMPLE DAILY CALORIC REQUIREMENT: 2,200*

EXAMPLE 1 | TOTAL CALORIES: 2,140

Breakfast
Steel Cut Oatmeal & Fruit: 330 Calories

Lunch
Caprese Salad with Burrata: 370 Calories

Snack
4 Hardboiled Eggs: 320 Calories

Dinner
Braised Beef with Tomatoes & Olives: 610 Calories

Dessert
Strawberry Ice Cream with Chocolate Sauce:
510 Calories

EXAMPLE 2 | TOTAL CALORIES: 2,140

Breakfast
Baked Eggs with Salsa Verde: 250 Calories

Lunch
Grilled Corn & Summer Vegetable Salad: 400 Calories
1 Piece of Fruit: 100 Calories

Snack
2 Easy Granola Bars: 520 Calories

Dinner
Green Bean Casserole: 220 Calories
Caramelized Brussels Sprouts: 170 Calories

Dessert
Chocolate Cake: 480 Calories

Based on the average calorie requirement for men, which varies depending on metabolism, exercise level, and other factors. Use a free online app to calculate your daily calorie needs.

Note: Men can follow the samples for women, as well. To increase the calories, add more walnuts to the first dessert, more dark chocolate and almonds to the second snack, and a bit of cheese to the second dessert.

WHAT TO EAT

All you need to know is the "Seven-Word Diet" from author Michael Pollan: "Eat food. Not too much. Mostly plants."

Okay, next chapter. Just kidding. But seriously, that's about as complex as it needs to be.

Fruits and Vegetables

Fruits and vegetables have a low glycemic load, meaning they'll help keep your blood sugar steady. They're loaded with fiber and nutrients. And quite frankly, people who eat more fruits and vegetables tend to eat less refined carbs.

Research has linked consumption of nutrient-dense foods, such as fruits and vegetables, with lower BMIs. In a large U.S. sample, overweight and obese people had lower intakes of dietary fiber (e.g., lentils, kale, mushrooms, spinach, and broccoli).[291] Meanwhile, they had more animal protein, meats, fats, and carbonated and sugar-sweetened beverages in their diet.

But in a weight loss study published in the *American Journal of Clinical Nutrition,* people who ate more fruits and vegetables—and that was the *only* difference between the two groups' diets—lost more weight after one year than the group that didn't increase their fruit and vegetable intake.[292] (Both groups had similar reductions in fat intake.) The fruit and vegetable group also reported feeling less hungry.

Fruits and vegetables are low calorie, keep you full longer, and are packed with nutrients. And, clearly, fruit won't make you fat. That's another myth. There's no need to balk at the sugar content of fruit if you're eating fresh, whole fruits: The fiber content slows the body's absorption of fructose, the main sugar content in fruit, so it enters the bloodstream slowly. There is not a single case of obesity in America due to eating too much whole fruit. I'll bet my reputation on that.

Nuts

Some people believe they should avoid nuts when trying to lose weight or that nuts will make them fat. It's not true! In fact, nuts are one of the three main components of my fat loss diet foundation (the other two are fruits and vegetables).

Not only is consumption of raw nuts believed to lower risk of heart disease, it can actually help you lose weight: Diets that include nuts have been linked with improved compliance (sticking with the diet) and greater weight loss compared with diets that forbid nuts.[293] Nut eaters often have a lower BMI than non-nut eaters.[294]

One weight loss study compared an almond-enriched diet to a complex-carb-enriched diet. Although both groups lost weight (because both food types are filling), the nut eaters had a sustained and greater reduction in fat.[295]

Raw nuts are a great source of fiber, healthy fats, and even a little protein. The key is sticking with raw nuts (rather than nuts roasted in oil or covered in sugar) and eating them in moderation. One of my favorite snacks—especially during my many travels around America—is an ounce (28 g) (or two [56 g], if I'm really hungry) of almonds, cashews, pecans, or walnuts.

Meat Is Fine

A healthy diet can include meat. Both the Mediterranean and low-carb diets, which often include meat, have proven more effective for weight loss than low-fat diets.[296]

A good rule of thumb is to choose high-quality protein (organic meats, wild-caught salmon, and cage-free eggs, for example).

In general, processed meats (such as deli meats, sausages, and fried meats) should be avoided. If your lunch includes a $1 burger from a value meal menu, chances are "quality" is not the first word a nutrition expert would use to describe it. When it comes to meat, you get what you pay for!

Water, Coffee, Tea, and (Sometimes) Wine

Drinking more water every day has been associated with weight loss *independent* of diet and physical activity.[297] I advocate for twelve cups (3 liters), consumed throughout the day and during exercise. Sparkling water is fine, too.

In addition to water, green tea, black tea, and black coffee (without added cream or sugar) are great calorie-free beverages.

Diet sodas are not recommended: They're loaded with chemicals that often make cravings worse, leading to calorie compensation in other food choices. However, if you were going to choose between a diet soda and regular soda, diet soda is still a better choice for weight loss, although neither could ever be called healthy.

The number of calories in the American diet has drastically increased compared with thirty years ago, and roughly *half* of the calorie increase takes the form of liquid calories—primarily sugar-sweetened drinks, such as juices and sodas. In one study, obese women reported drinking the highest amount of sugar-sweetened and carbonated beverages across all sex and BMI categories.[298] Clearly, avoiding beverages that contain calories is an important, and easy, solution for weight loss.

The number of calories in the American diet has drastically increased compared with thirty years ago, and roughly half *of the calorie increase takes the form of liquid calories—primarily sugar-sweetened drinks, such as juices and sodas.*

Alcoholic drinks are also loaded with calories, and studies show that beyond one to two drinks a day, the heart health benefits seem to disappear.[299] Every once in a while, I'll have a drink with dinner, but I pretty much left alcohol behind in my frat boy days.

For many people, minimizing or completely eliminating alcohol intake is the healthiest choice and another easy way to cut back on calories and speed fat loss.

In a nutshell: Drink water, tea, and plain coffee; skip juices, sodas, and diet sodas.

WHAT NOT TO EAT

We've already seen what not to eat, but it bears repeating: No added sugars; no processed carbs. They will not help you reach your goals and are counterproductive at the very least. Let's look closer.

Added Sugar

In 2004, the average American ate 22.2 teaspoons (89 g)—or 355 calories—of added sugars per day.[300] The American Heart Association recommends half that: one hundred calories of added sugar for women and 150 for men, at a *maximum*. If you're eating a lot of added sugars, cutting back will accelerate fat loss and improve your heart health.

Soda is easily the worst added-sugar offender, and per-person daily consumption of soda has risen more than 70 percent since the 1970s, up to 13.2 ounces (390 ml) a day.[301]

A report from the Nurses' Health Study showed that women who consumed diets with a high glycemic load, related to eating lots of highly processed starches and sweets, had an increased risk of coronary heart disease.[302] When researchers followed up with this group after ten years, those with the highest consumption of high glycemic index foods had *double* the risk of those in the lowest-consumption group.

What is added sugar? It's the sugars and syrups added to processed and prepared foods in alarming amounts, as well as whatever you heap into your food and drinks from the sugar bowl on the table. The lion's share of the added sugar consumption in the United States can be found in soft drinks, fruit drinks, desserts, candy, and boxed cereals.[303]

And yes, added sugar includes all the crazy names it can be disguised as . . . especially now that "cane syrup," "agave nectar," and "brown rice syrup" are showing up in so-called healthy or organic drinks.

Processed Carbs

A diet high in refined carbohydrates (such as white flour) poses a number of health risks. But that's exactly the kind of diet lots of people follow when they hear the "low-fat, high-carb" recommendations from health organizations.[304]

Processed carbohydrates increase insulin, lead to fat storage, and do not result in satiety . . . thus you get hungry fast.[305] People have developed more food addictions around processed foods high in carbs than any other food group.

Furthermore, refined carbs have barely any nutritional value. The fiber and other nutrients (such as B-complex vitamins and healthy oils) have all been removed.

SIX KEYS TO SUCCESS

Adopting these habits will make healthy eating simpler and easier than any diet:

1. **Edit your environment.** Keep the junk out of the house and out of your desk at work—or at least, keep it hidden! Research shows we eat what's in plain sight. Place healthy snacks—fruits, vegetables, raw nuts—in plain view (like in fruit bowls on your kitchen counter). Another important part of your environment is social: Lean on others for support to help you stick with your healthy eating goals and steer clear of social situations if the food temptations will be too difficult to handle. (Rituals like chewing gum or taking the dog for a quick walk can also help thwart binge eating.)

2. **Ditch the "cardio confessional."** If you binge on junk food at one meal, you can't make it disappear with a workout the next day. Rather than trying to "burn off" unhealthy food or excessive calories with a visit to the "cardio confessional"

(or an HIIT confessional, for that matter), stick with the 90–10 rule instead.

3. **Follow the 90–10 rule.** My friend John Berardi, Ph.D., introduced me to this superior way of eating compared with counting calories. The idea is simple: Allow 10 percent of your food to come from rewards or special meals and stick to your healthy eating plan the rest of the time. It has always worked for me.

4. **Take baby steps.** Most people, like Catherine, jump into extreme and restrictive diets. It's no surprise they don't work. That's why I had her take a simpler approach: Start small with nutrition and exercise changes and continue to improve each week. The baby-step method can be as simple as committing to one small change every day and one big change per week.

For example, today you might have your coffee black instead of adding cream and sugar; tomorrow, you'll swap your afternoon soda for green tea or water. Other simple changes to make include shopping at a weekend farmers' market and then planning and preparing your meals for the coming week or trying a new vegetable at dinner every night this week.

Building your food and exercise foundation at a comfortable pace will help you avoid bad food binges. And trust me: One small daily change and one big weekly change will give you huge improvements in your energy, weight loss, and fitness results over time.

5. **Plan and prep.** By planning ahead and preparing your meals at home, you won't be tempted to visit the local fast-food joint because you didn't bring a lunch, and you'll also be less likely to give in to sudden cravings for junk food.

6. **Keep a food journal.** Record your daily eating habits: what you ate, how much, and when. You can, or don't have to, include calories. You might also record how you were feeling and what cravings you experienced. Being aware of your food intake and your behaviors can help you make healthier decisions about your diet.

Eating high-quality whole foods may be a little more expensive than buying junk food, but, at the end of the day, if diet is even more important than exercise, and exercise—no matter how short—involves hard work, isn't it worth making all your hard work count?

SIX KEYS TO SUCCESS

Remember: If you follow these six habits, you'll never need to go near a diet again.

1. Edit your environment.
2. Ditch the "cardio confessional."
3. Follow the 90–10 rule.
4. Take baby steps.
5. Plan and prep.
6. Keep a food journal.

FURTHER RESOURCES

www.cardiomythweightloss.com
Here you'll find the latest exercise and nutrition advice from Craig, including new workouts, recipes, and daily challenges.

www.earlytorise.com
Craig is also a Productivity & Success Transformation Coach. On ETR, he teaches men and women how to use his 5 Pillars of Transformation and other principles to get the body of their dreams, get a raise and make more money, find the love of their life, and overcome any obstacle in the way of success.

www.homeworkoutrevolution.com
In 2013, Craig released the Home Workout Revolution bodyweight exercise program, complete with 51 no-equipment home workouts and accompanying instructional videos.

www.turbulencetraining.com
Craig created this popular home workout program in 2001 and it's still going strong. Check out the official site to learn more about the Turbulence Training Program and view success stories.

GLOSSARY

Aerobic activity: This is an activity that requires consuming a lot of oxygen over a continuous period of time (e.g., steady-state cardio).

Anaerobic activity: This is an activity that requires short bursts of higher exertion, with an individual running out of breath fairly quickly (e.g., HIIT and strength training).

Body composition: This describes proportions of lean mass and fat mass in the body. Because muscle weighs more than fat, a better goal than weight loss is improvement in body composition—that is, a decrease in excess body fat and/or an increase in muscle. Exercise studies should measure changes in body fat mass and inches, not just weight.

Body mass index (BMI): This is a ratio of height to weight. While not an accurate indicator of body fat percentage, there is often a correlation between body fat and BMI, unless a person has a lot of muscle. In general, a BMI of 18.5–24.9 is considered healthy, while 25–29.9 is classified as overweight, and 30 or higher is obese.

Calorie: This is a unit used to measure energy; for example, the potential energy that a food product gives us. If we consume more energy than our body uses, it gets stored in the body and we gain weight. So, when a machine or monitor tells you how many calories you're burning, this is a proxy for how much energy it thinks you're using.

Cardio: This term generally refers to aerobic exercise done at a steady or continuous pace, usually sustained for a longer period of time (e.g., 20 minutes or more). It's sometimes called endurance activity or steady-state cardio. Examples include cycling, running, walking, and using elliptical machines.

Cardio confessional: This is a term I use for the (misguided) belief that a person can reverse a bad diet and other unhealthy lifestyle choices through extra cardio exercise.

Cardiovascular disease (CVD): There are two types of cardiovascular disease: coronary (ischemic) heart disease and cerebrovascular heart disease. In addition to genetic predisposition and previously existing conditions, coronary heart disease risk is more heavily influenced by lifestyle behaviors, including diet, stress levels, physical activity, and whether one consumes tobacco or alcohol.

Compensation effect: Engaging in exercise leads some individuals to compensate unconsciously for energy expended by increasing daily caloric intake or reducing non-exercise physical activity. This tendency can hinder fat loss efforts.

Energy expenditure: At its simplest level, this is the total amount of energy, or calories, your body uses each day or to perform a specific activity.

Fat-burning zone: This is the theory that optimal fat-burning results come from exercise in a zone of low, rather than high, intensity. This has been disproven by research demonstrating the potential for HIIT to cause superior fat loss compared to steady-state cardio.

Female athlete triad: This is a group of inter-related conditions (amenorrhea, brittle bones, and disordered eating) caused by insufficient nutrition relative to physical exertion. These can harm reproductive health, increase risk of bone fractures, and, in some cases, be fatal.

High-intensity interval training (HIIT): This is exercise that alternates short bursts of anaerobic activity and very low-intensity aerobic activity. Also called high-intensity intermittent exercise (HIIE), this type of exercise can be done with either a cardio activity (e.g., cycling) or a resistance activity (e.g., bodyweight circuits).

Metabolic syndrome: This is a group of factors that increases the risk of diabetes, coronary heart disease, and stroke. These factors include abdominal obesity (i.e., visceral fat), high blood pressure, a high triglyceride level, and insulin resistance.

Metabolism: How much energy, or calories, your body requires to perform daily tasks is called your metabolism. Basal metabolic rate, or resting metabolic rate, accounts for roughly 70 percent of a person's daily calorie expenditure and refers to the number of calories the body uses "at rest" for basic functions, such as blood circulation and the growth and repair of cells. It is influenced by genetics, body size and composition, and, to a lesser extent, physical activity. Exercise and thermogenesis (digesting food) also comprise a portion of daily calorie expenditure. Muscle mass is the biggest contributor to metabolic rate.

Resistance exercise: Also called strength training, it uses movements with added resistance, created either with weights or a person's bodyweight. Some newer HIIT protocols incorporate strength exercises with interval cardio, and some are even completely resistance-focused.

Skinny fat: This describes having a small, but weak and flabby, physique due to muscle loss. It can be caused by years (or even just months) of endurance exercise with no strength training.

Subcutaneous fat: This is the fat above the muscles. It tends to accumulate around the thighs, upper arms, belly, and waist (e.g., "love handles").

Visceral fat: This is the belly fat below the stomach muscles that is linked with increased risk of cardiovascular disease and type 2 diabetes. Visceral fat accumulation can be reversed or prevented with diet, as well as exercises that promote fat loss.

VO2max: This is a measure of cardiovascular fitness used in scientific research studies. It reflects a person's maximal oxygen uptake during exercise. A simpler way to gauge intensity can be found in chapters 4 and 8.

REFERENCES

1   Utter, A.C., Nieman, D.C., Shannonhouse, E.M., Butterworth, D.E., & Nieman, C.N. (1998). Influence of diet and/or exercise on body composition and cardiorespiratory fitness in obese women. *International Journal of Sport Nutrition, 8*(3), 213–222.

2   Redman, L.M., Heilbronn, L.K., Martin, C.K., Alfonso, A., Smith, S.R., & Ravussin, E. (2007). Effect of calorie restriction with or without exercise on body composition and fat distribution. *The Journal of Clinical Endocrinology & Metabolism, 92*(3), 865–872.

3   McTiernan, A., Sorensen, B., Irwin, M.L., Morgan, A., Yasui, Y., Rudolph, R.E., . . . Potter, J.D. (2007). Exercise effect on weight and body fat in men and women. *Obesity, 15*(6), 1496–1512.

4   Fothergill, E., Guo, J., Howard, L., Kerns, J.C., Knuth, N.D., Brychta, R., . . . & Hall, K.D. (2016). Persistent metabolic adaptation 6 years after "The Biggest Loser" competition. *Obesity, 24*(8), 1612–1619.

5   Kolata, G. (2016, May 2). After "The Biggest Loser," their bodies fought to regain weight. *New York Times*. Retrieved from: www.nytimes.com/2016/05/02/health/biggest-loser-weight-loss.html

6   Reynolds, G. (2014, December 10). Got a minute? Let's work out. *New York Times*. Retrieved from: http://well.blogs.nytimes.com/2014/12/10/one-minute-workout

7   Kennedy, J.F. (1960). The soft American. *Sports Illustrated, 13*(26), 14–17.

8   Reinhold, R. (1987, March 29). An interview with Kenneth Cooper. *New York Times*, Late Edition (East Coast): A.14.

9   Cooper Aerobics. (n.d.). *About*. Retrieved from: www.cooperaerobics.com/About.aspx

10   Ibid.

11   Cooper, K.H., Pollock, M.L., Martin, R. P., White, S.R., Linnerud, A.C., & Jackson, A. (1976). Physical fitness levels vs. selected coronary risk factors: a cross-sectional study. *JAMA, 236*(2), 166–169.

12   Blair, S.N., Kohl, H.W., Paffenbarger, R.S., Clark, D.G., Cooper, K.H., & Gibbons, L.W. (1989). Physical fitness and all-cause mortality: a prospective study of healthy men and women. *JAMA, 262*(17), 2395–2401.

13   Young, S. (1978, October 14). Books the aerobics way by Kenneth H. Cooper, M.D. *The Globe and Mail* (Toronto, Ontario), S.18.

14   McDowell, E. (1982, December 15). How the public received an important message. *The Globe and Mail* (Toronto, Ontario), P.15.

15   Feineman, N. (1986, February 23). Exercise pays off, father of aerobics says: Cooper looks at fitness in the '80s. *Chicago Sun-Times* (Chicago, Illinois): 13; Williams, J. Cooper. (1988, July 29). First word in aerobics / fitness "father" still in

forefront of health crusade. The Tribune (San Diego, California): D2; Slovut, G. (1989, March 25). Aerobics champion has run 23,500 miles in quest for fitness. *Star Tribune* (Minneapolis, Minnesota): 01E.

16 Reinhold. (1987, March 29). *New York Times*, Late Edition (East Coast): A.14.

17 Ibid.

18 Slovut. (1989, March 25). *Star Tribune*: 01E.

19 Running USA. (n.d.). Retrieved from: www.runningusa.org/statistics

20 Statista. (2015). Number of joggers and runners in the U.S.A. Retrieved from: www.statista.com/statistics/227423/number-of-joggers-and-runners-usa

21 Centers for Disease Control, National Center for Health Statistics. (2016). Obesity and overweight. Retrieved from: www.cdc.gov/nchs/fastats/obesity-overweight.htm

22 Schroeder, S.A. (2007). We can do better—improving the health of the American people. *New England Journal of Medicine*, 357(12), 1221–1228.

23 Ibid.

24 National Center for Chronic Disease Prevention and Health Promotion, Division for Heart Disease and Stroke Prevention. (2015). *Heart disease facts*. Retrieved from: www.cdc.gov/heartdisease/facts.htm

25 American Psychological Association. (2014). Stress snapshot. Retrieved from: www.apa.org/news/press/releases/stress/2014/snapshot.aspx

26 McTiernan, Sorensen, Irwin, Morgan, Yasui, Rudolph, . . . Potter. (2007). *Obesity*, 15(6), 1496–1512.

27 Trapp, E.G., Chisholm, D.J., Freund, J., & Boutcher, S.H. (2008). The effects of high-intensity intermittent exercise training on fat loss and fasting insulin levels of young women. *International Journal of Obesity*, 32(4), 684–691.

28 Tan, M., Fat, R.C.M., Boutcher, Y.N., & Boutcher S.H. (2014). Effect of high-intensity intermittent exercise on postprandial plasma triacylglycerol in sedentary young women. *International Journal of Sport Nutrition and Exercise Metabolism*, 24(1), 110–18.

29 King, N.A., Hopkins, M., Caudwell, P., Stubbs, R.J., & Blundell, J.E. (2008). Individual variability following twelve weeks of supervised exercise: identification and characterization of compensation for exercise-induced weight loss. *International Journal of Obesity*, 32(1), 177–184.

30 Centers for Disease Control and Prevention, National Center for Health Statistics. (2014, September). Prevalence of overweight, obesity, and extreme obesity among adults: United States, 1960–1962 through 2011–2012. Retrieved from: ww.cdc.gov/nchs/data/hestat/obesity_adult_11_12/obesity_adult_11_12.htm

31 Louie, E. (1981, August 30). Working out. *New York Times*, Late Edition (East Coast): A.238.

32 Janssen, G.M., Graef, C.J., & Saris, W.H. (1989). Food intake and body composition in novice athletes during a training period to run a marathon. *International Journal of Sports Medicine*, 10(suppl 1), S17–21.

33 Paffenbarger Jr, R.S., & Hale, W.E. (1975). Work activity and coronary heart mortality. *New England Journal of Medicine*, 292(11), 545–550.

34 Taylor, H.L., Klepetar, E., Keys, A., Parlin, W., Blackburn, H., & Puchner, T. (1962). Death rates among physically active and sedentary employees of the railroad industry. *American Journal of Public Health and the Nation's Health*, 52(10), 1697–1707.

35 Tremblay, A., Simoneau, J.A., & Bouchard, C. (1994). Impact of exercise intensity on body fatness and skeletal muscle metabolism. *Metabolism*, 43(7), 814–818.

36　Boutcher, S.H. (2010). High-intensity intermittent exercise and fat loss. *Journal of Obesity, 2011*. doi: 10.1155/2011/868305

37　Polley, M. (1981). *Dance Aerobics*. New York: Anderson World.

38　Thompson, H. (1995, June). Walk, don't run. *Texas Monthly*. Retrieved from: www.texasmonthly.com/articles/walk-dont-run

39　U.S. Department of Health and Human Services. (n.d.). Office of Disease Prevention and Health Promotion. Healthy People 2020. *Physical activity*. Retrieved from: www.healthypeople.gov/2020/topics-objectives/topic/physical-activity

40　Mayo Clinic Staff. (2014, November 15). Exercise for weight loss: Calories burned in 1 hour. Retrieved from: www.mayoclinic.org/healthy-lifestyle/weight-loss/in-depth/exercise/art-20050999

41　Wu, T., Gao, X., Chen, M., & Van Dam, R.M. (2009). Long-term effectiveness of diet-plus-exercise interventions versus diet-only interventions for weight loss: a meta-analysis. *Obesity Reviews, 10*(3), 313–323.

42　Florida Atlantic University. (2013, January 31). Obesity approaching cigarette smoking as leading avoidable cause of premature deaths worldwide. *ScienceDaily*. Retrieved from: www.sciencedaily.com/releases/2013/01/130131083755.htm

43　World Health Organization. (n.d.). Physical inactivity: a global public health problem. *Global Strategy on Diet, Physical Activity, and Health*. Retrieved from: www.who.int/dietphysicalactivity/factsheet_inactivity/en/

44　Poirier, P., Giles, T.D., Bray, G.A., Hong, Y., Stern, J.S., Pi-Sunyer, F.X., & Eckel, R.H. (2006). Obesity and cardiovascular disease: pathophysiology, evaluation, and effect of weight loss. An update of the 1997 American Heart Association scientific statement on obesity and heart disease from the obesity committee of the council on nutrition, physical activity, and metabolism. *Circulation, 113*(6), 898–918.

45　Wyatt, S.B., Winters, K.P., & Dubbert, P.M. (2006). Overweight and obesity: prevalence, consequences, and causes of a growing public health problem. *The American Journal of the Medical Sciences, 331*(4), 166–174.

46　Bauer, U.E., Briss, P.A., Goodman, R.A., & Bowman, B.A. (2014). Prevention of chronic disease in the twenty-first century: elimination of the leading preventable causes of premature death and disability in the U.S.A. *The Lancet, 384*(9937), 45–52.

47　United States Department of Agriculture. (2002). Profiling food consumption in America. *Agriculture fact book, chapter 2*. Retrieved from: www.usda.gov/factbook/chapter2.pdf

48　Chaput, J.P., Després, J.P., Bouchard, C., & Tremblay, A. (2008). The association between sleep duration and weight gain in adults: a six-year prospective study from the Quebec Family Study. *Sleep, 31*(4), 517–523.

49　Wyatt, Winters, & Dubbert. (2006). *The American Journal of the Medical Sciences, 331*(4), 166–174.

50　Boutcher. (2010). *Journal of Obesity*, 2011.

51　Tremblay, A., Després, J. P., Leblanc, C., Craig, C. L., Ferris, B., Stephens, T., & Bouchard, C. (1990). Effect of intensity of physical activity on body fatness and fat distribution. *The American Journal of Clinical Nutrition, 51*(2), 153–157.

52　Tremblay, Simoneau, & Bouchard. (1994). *Metabolism, 43*(7), 814–818.

53　Boutcher. (2010). *Journal of Obesity, 2011*.

54　Trapp, Chisholm, Freund, & Boutcher. (2008). *International Journal of Obesity, 32*(4), 684–691.

55   Irving, B.A., Davis, C.K., Brock, D.W., Weltman, J.Y., Swift, D., Barrett, E.J., . . . Weltman, A. (2008). Effect of exercise training intensity on abdominal visceral fat and body composition. *Medicine & Science in Sports & Exercise*, *40*(11), 1863–1872.

56   Bryner, R.W., Ullrich, I.H., Sauers, J., Donley, D., Hornsby, G., Kolar, M., & Yeater, R. (1999). Effects of resistance vs. aerobic training combined with an 800 calorie liquid diet on lean body mass and resting metabolic rate. *Journal of the American College of Nutrition*, *18*(2), 115–121.

57   Park, S.K., Park, J.H., Kwon, Y.C., Kim, H.S., Yoon, M.S., & Park, I.I.T. (2003). The effect of combined aerobic and resistance exercise training on abdominal fat in obese middle-aged women. *Journal of Physiological Anthropology and Applied Human Science*, *22*(3), 129–135.

58   Wyatt, Winters, & Dubbert. (2006). *The American Journal of the Medical Sciences*, *331*(4), 166–174.

59   Ibid.

60   Field, A.E., Coakley, E.H., Must, A., Spadano, J.L., Laird, N., Dietz, W.H., . . . Colditz, G.A. (2001). Impact of overweight on the risk of developing common chronic diseases during a 10-year period. *Archives of Internal Medicine*, *161*(13), 1581–1586.

61   Harvard Health Publications. (2005, September 1). Abdominal fat and what to do about it. *The Family Health Guide*. Retrieved from: www.health.harvard.edu/staying-healthy/abdominal-fat-and-what-to-do-about-it

62   Ibid.

63   Ibid.

64   Centers for Disease Control, National Center for Chronic Disease Prevention and Health Promotion, Division of Nutrition, Physical Activity, and Obesity. (2015, May). *Physical activity for a healthy weight*. Retrieved from: www.cdc.gov/healthyweight/physical_activity/index.html

65   Office of Disease Prevention and Health Promotion. (2016, May). Physical activity guidelines for Americans. Retrieved from: http://health.gov/PAGuidelines/guidelines

66   McTiernan, Sorensen, Irwin, Morgan, Yasui, Rudolph, . . . & Potter. (2007). *Obesity*, *15*(6), 1496–1512.

67   King, Hopkins, Caudwell, Stubbs, & Blundell. (2008). *International Journal of Obesity*, *32*(1), 177–184.

68   Boutcher, & Dunn. (2009). *Obesity Reviews*, *10*(6), 671–680.

69   Janssen, Graef, & Saris. (1989). *International Journal of Sports Medicine*, *10*(suppl 1), S17–21.

70   King, Hopkins, Caudwell, Stubbs, & Blundell. (2008). *International Journal of Obesity*, *32*(1), 177–184.

71   Boutcher, & Dunn. (2009). *Obesity Reviews*, *10*(6), 671–680.

72   Zelman, K. (2005, July 26). Are the sexes really different when it comes to losing weight? *WebMD Feature Archive*. Retrieved from: www.webmd.com/diet/weight-loss-wars-men-vs-women.

73   Fell, J. (2011, May 16). The myth of ripped muscles and calorie burns. *Los Angeles Times*. Retrieved from: http://articles.latimes.com/2011/may/16/health/la-he-fitness-muscle-myth-20110516

74   Trapp, Chisholm, Freund, & Boutcher. (2008). *International Journal of Obesity*, *32*(4), 684–691.

75   Centers for Disease Control and Prevention, National Center for Health Statistics. (2015, June). Health, United States, 2014 *NCHS FACT SHEET*. Retrieved from: www.cdc.gov/nchs/data/factsheets/factsheet_health_us.htm

76   Polley, M. (1981). *Dance Aerobics*.

77   Nsubuga, J. (2015, July 21). Sir David Frost's son dies after collapsing while jogging. *MetroUK*. Retrieved from: http://metro.co.uk/2015/07/21/sir-david-frosts-son-dies-after-collapsing-while-jogging-5305427

78   Logan, W.P.D. (1952). Mortality from coronary and myocardial disease in different social classes. *The Lancet, 259*(6711), 758–759.

79   Morris, J.N., Heady, J.A., Raffle, P.A.B., Roberts, C.G., & Parks, J.W. (1953). Coronary heart-disease and physical activity of work. *The Lancet, 262*(6796), 1111–1120.

80   Ibid.

81   Fox 3rd, S.M., & Haskell, W.L. (1968). Physical activity and the prevention of coronary heart disease. *Bulletin of the New York Academy of Medicine, 44*(8), 950–965.

82   Paffenbarger Jr, & Hale. (1975). *New England Journal of Medicine, 292*(11), 545–550.

83   Mosca, L., Barrett-Connor, E., & Wenger, N.K. (2011). Sex/gender differences in cardiovascular disease prevention: what a difference a decade makes. *Circulation, 124*(19), 2145–2154.

84   Mehta, L.S., Beckie, T.M., DeVon, H.A., Grines, C.L., Krumholz, H.M., Johnson, M.N., . . . Wenger, N.K. (2016). Acute myocardial infarction in women: a scientific statement from the American Heart Association. *Circulation, 133*(9), 916–947.

85   Stampfer, M.J., Hu, F.B., Manson, J.E., Rimm, E.B., & Willett, W.C. (2000). Primary prevention of coronary heart disease in women through diet and lifestyle. *New England Journal of Medicine, 343*(1), 16–22.

86   Leepson, M. (1978). Physical fitness boom. *Editorial Research Reports 1978* (Vol. I). Washington, D.C.: CQ Press. Retrieved from: http://library.cqpress.com/cqresearcher/cqresrre1978041400

87   Bassler, T.J. (1977). Marathon running and immunity to atherosclerosis. *Annals of the New York Academy of Sciences, 301*(1), 579–592.

88   Waller, B.F., & Roberts, W.C. (1980). Sudden death while running in conditioned runners aged 40 years or over. *The American Journal of Cardiology, 45*(6), 1292–1300.

89   Robbins, J. (2011, January 31). What should we learn from the deaths of fitness icons? *The Huffington Post*. Retrieved from: www.huffingtonpost.com/john-robbins/what-should-we-learn-from_b_815943.html

90   O'Keefe, J.H., Schnohr, P., & Lavie, C.J. (2013). The dose of running that best confers longevity. *Heart, 99*(8), 588–590.

91   Webner, D., Drezner, J., Horneff, J., & Roberts, W. (2011). Sudden cardiac arrest and death in United States marathons. *British Journal of Sports Medicine, 45*(4), 315–316.

92   Marijon, E., Tafflet, M., Celermajer, D.S., Dumas, F., Perier, M.C., Mustafic, H., . . . Jouven, X. (2011). Sports-related sudden death in the general population. *Circulation, 124*(6), 672–681.

93   Mehta, Beckie, DeVon, Grines, Krumholz, Johnson, . . . & Wenger. (2016). *Circulation, 133*(9), 916–947.

94   Shmerling, R. (2016, February 19). Why men often die earlier than women. *Harvard Health Publications*. Retrieved from: www.health.harvard.edu/blog/why-men-often-die-earlier-than-women-201602199137

95   Robbins, J. (2011, January 31). *The Huffington Post*.

96   Hill, D. (2010, September 21). Raising the power bar: the Brian Maxwell story. *Canadian Running*. Retrieved from: http://runningmagazine.ca/raising-the-power-bar-the-brian-maxwell-story

97   Altman, L. (1984, July 24). The doctor's world; James Fixx: the enigma of heart disease. *New York Times*. Retrieved from: www.nytimes.com/1984/07/24/science/the-doctor-s-world-james-fixx-the-enigma-of-heart-disease.html

98   World Health Organization. (2015, January). Cardiovascular diseases (CVDs). *Fact sheet*. Retrieved from: www.who.int/mediacentre/factsheets/fs317/en/

99   Arango, T. (2016, February 3). Baghdad hosts a 'marathon' and celebrates a victory. *New York Times*. Retrieved from: www.nytimes.com/2016/02/04/world/middleeast/baghdad-international-marathon.html

100   World Health Organization. (2015, January). *Fact sheet*.

101   American Heart Association. (2014, April). Atherosclerosis. Retrieved from: www.heart.org/HEARTORG/Conditions/Cholesterol/WhyCholesterolMatters/Atherosclerosis_UCM_305564_Article.jsp#.V1T3FOcrK2w

102   Fox 3rd, & Haskell. (1968). *Bulletin of the New York Academy of Medicine, 44*(8), 950.

103   National Heart, Lung, and Blood Institute. (2014, April 21). Who is at risk for heart disease? Retrieved from: www.nhlbi.nih.gov/health/health-topics/topics/hdw/atrisk

104   Fox 3rd, & Haskell. (1968). *Bulletin of the New York Academy of Medicine, 44*(8), 950.

105   O'Keefe, Schnohr, & Lavie. (2013). *Heart, 99*(8), 588–590.

106   Stampfer, Hu, Manson, Rimm, & Willett. (2000). *New England Journal of Medicine, 343*(1), 16–22.

107   Mosca, Barrett-Connor, & Wenger. (2011). *Circulation, 124*(19), 2145–2154.

108   Kannel, W.B., & Sorlie, P. (1979). Some health benefits of physical activity. The Framingham study. *Archives of Internal Medicine, 139*(8), 857–861.

109   Stampfer, Hu, Manson, Rimm, & Willett. (2000). *New England Journal of Medicine, 343*(1), 16–22.

110   Feineman, Neil. (1986, February 23). Exercise pays off, father of aerobics says: Cooper looks at fitness in the '80s. *Chicago Sun-Times*, p. 13.

111   Boehm, J.K., & Kubzansky, L.D. (2012). The heart's content: the association between positive psychological well-being and cardiovascular health. *Psychological Bulletin, 138*(4), 655–691.

112   Fox 3rd, & Haskell. (1968). *Bulletin of the New York Academy of Medicine, 44*(8), 950.

113   National Heart, Lung, and Blood Institute. (n.d.). Assessing your weight and health risk. Retrieved from: www.nhlbi.nih.gov/health/educational/lose_wt/risk.htm

114   Warburton, D.E., Nicol, C.W., & Bredin, S.S. (2006). Health benefits of physical activity: the evidence. *Canadian Medical Association Journal, 174*(6), 801–809.

115   Braith, R.W., & Stewart, K.J. (2006). Resistance exercise training its role in the prevention of cardiovascular disease. *Circulation, 113*(22), 2642–2650.

116   Pierson, L.M., Herbert, W.G., Norton, H.J., Kiebzak, G.M., Griffith, P., Fedor, J.M., . . . Cook, J.W. (2001). Effects of combined aerobic and resistance training versus aerobic training alone in cardiac rehabilitation. *Journal of Cardiopulmonary Rehabilitation and Prevention, 21*(2), 101–110.

117   Paffenbarger Jr, & Hale. (1975). *New England Journal of Medicine, 292*(11), 545–550.

118   Reinhold. (1987, March 29). *New York Times*, Late Edition (East Coast): A.14.

119 Solomon, H.A. (1984). *The Exercise Myth*. New York: Harcourt Brace Jovanovich.

120 Marijon, E., Tafflet, M., Celermajer, D. S., Dumas, F., Perier, M.C., Mustafic, H., . . . Jouven, X. (2011). Sports-related sudden death in the general population. *Circulation, 124*(6), 672–681.

121 Solomon. (1984). *The Exercise Myth*.

122 Schnohr, P., O'Keefe, J.H., Marott, J.L., Lange, P., & Jensen, G.B. (2015). Dose of jogging and long-term mortality: the Copenhagen city heart study. *Journal of the American College of Cardiology, 65*(5), 411–419.

123 Eijsvogels, T.M., Molossi, S., Lee, D.C., Emery, M.S., & Thompson, P.D. (2016). Exercise at the extremes: the amount of exercise to reduce cardiovascular events. *Journal of the American College of Cardiology, 67*(3), 316–329.

124 O'Keefe, Schnohr, & Lavie. (2013). *Heart, 99*(8), 588–590.

125 Schnohr, O'Keefe, Marott, Lange, & Jensen. (2015). *Journal of the American College of Cardiology, 65*(5), 411–419.

126 Chugh, S.S., & Weiss, J.B. (2015). Sudden cardiac death in the older athlete. *Journal of the American College of Cardiology, 65*(5), 493–502.

127 O'Keefe, Schnohr, & Lavie. (2013). *Heart, 99*(8), 588–590.

128 Ibid.

129 Ibid.

130 Ophir, E., Nass, C., & Wagner, A.D. (2009). Cognitive control in media multitaskers. *Proceedings of the National Academy of Sciences, 106*(37), 15583–15587.

131 Statista. (2016). Digital ad spending: U.S. consumer electronics industry 2011–2017. Retrieved from: www.statista.com/statistics/235941/us-consumer-electronics-industry-online-ad-spending

132 Governors Highway Safety Association. (2016, May). Distracted driving laws. Retrieved from: www.ghsa.org/html/stateinfo/laws/cellphone_laws.html

133 Redelmeier, D.A., & Tibshirani, R.J. (1997). Association between cellular-telephone calls and motor vehicle collisions. *New England Journal of Medicine, 336*(7), 453–458.

134 Strayer, D.L., Drews, F.A., & Crouch, D.J. (2006). A comparison of the cell phone driver and the drunk driver. *Human Factors: The Journal of the Human Factors and Ergonomics Society, 48*(2), 381–391.

135 Dahl, M. (2010, January). Gym-goers trip, flip and fall in pursuit of fitness. *Today.com*. Retrieved from: www.nbcnews.com/id/35127528/ns/health-fitness/t/gym-goers-trip-flip-fall-pursuit-fitness

136 Mayo Clinic. (2014, September 19). Metabolism and weight loss: how you burn calories. *Healthy Lifestyle*. Retrieved from: www.mayoclinic.org/healthy-lifestyle/weight-loss/in-depth/metabolism/art-20046508

137 University of Illinois, McKinley Health Center. (2016, May 10). Breaking down your metabolism. Retrieved from: www.mckinley.illinois.edu/handouts/metabolism.htm.

138 McTiernan, Sorensen, Irwin, Morgan, Yasui, Rudolph, . . . Potter. (2007). *Obesity, 15*(6), 1496–1512.

139 Garrow, J.S., & Summerbell, C.D. (1995). Meta-analysis: effect of exercise, with or without dieting, on the body composition of overweight subjects. *European Journal of Clinical Nutrition, 49*(1), 1–10.

140 Tremblay, Després, Leblanc, Craig, Ferris, Stephens, & Bouchard, C. (1990). *The American Journal of Clinical Nutrition, 51*(2), 153–157.

141 Irving, Davis, Brock, Weltman, Swift, Barrett, . . . Weltman. (2008). *Medicine & Science in Sports & Exercise*, *40*(11), 1863.

142 Trapp, Chisholm, Freund, & Boutcher. (2008). *International Journal of Obesity*, *32*(4), 684–691.

143 Tremblay, Simoneau, & Bouchard. (1994). *Metabolism*, *43*(7), 814–818.

144 Heydari, M., Freund, J., & Boutcher, S.H. (2012). The effect of high-intensity intermittent exercise on body composition of overweight young males. *Journal of Obesity, 2012*. doi: 10.1155/2012/480467

145 Logan, G.R., Harris, N., Duncan, S., Plank, L.D., Merien, F., & Schofield, G. (2016). Low-active male adolescents: a dose response to high-intensity interval training. *Medicine & Science in Sports & Exercise*, *48*(3), 481–490.

146 Pontzer, H., Durazo-Arvizu, R., Dugas, L.R., Plange-Rhule, J., Bovet, P., Forrester, T.E., . . . Luke, A. (2016). Constrained total energy expenditure and metabolic adaptation to physical activity in adult humans. *Current Biology*, *26*(3), 410–417.

147 Pontzer, H., Raichlen, D.A., Wood, B.M., Mabulla, A.Z., Racette, S.B., & Marlowe, F.W. (2012). Hunter–gatherer energetics and human obesity. *PLoS One*, *7*(7), e40503.

148 Pontzer, H. (2012, August 24). Debunking the hunter–gatherer workout. *New York Times*. Retrieved from: www.nytimes.com/2012/08/26/opinion/sunday/debunking-the-hunter-gatherer-workout.html

149 Khazan, O. (2016, April). Exercise in futility. *The Atlantic*. Retrieved from: www.theatlantic.com/magazine/archive/2016/04/exercise-in-futility/471492/

150 Wu, Gao, Chen, & Van Dam. (2009). *Obesity Reviews*, *10*(3), 313–323.

151 Garrow, & Summerbell. (1995). *European Journal of Clinical Nutrition*, *49*(1), 1–10.

152 Nicklas, B.J., Wang, X., You, T., Lyles, M.F., Demons, J., Easter, L., . . . Carr, J.J. (2009). Effect of exercise intensity on abdominal fat loss during calorie restriction in overweight and obese postmenopausal women: a randomized, controlled trial. *The American Journal of Clinical Nutrition*, *89*(4), 1043–1052.

153 Foster, G.D., Wadden, T.A., Kendrick, Z.V., Letizia, K.A., Lander, D.P., & Conill, A.M. (1995). The energy cost of walking before and after significant weight loss. *Medicine & Science in Sports & Exercise*, *27*(6), 888–894.

154 Saris, W.H., Blair, S.N., van Baak, M.A., Eaton, S.B., Davies, P.S., Di Pietro, L., . . . Wyatt, H. (2003). How much physical activity is enough to prevent unhealthy weight gain? Outcome of the IASO 1st stock conference and consensus statement. *Obesity Reviews*, *4*(2), 101–114.

155 Shaw, K.A., Gennat, H.C., O'Rourke, P., & Del Mar, C. (2006). Exercise for overweight or obesity. *The Cochrane Library*, (4): CD003817.

156 Irving, Davis, Brock, Weltman, Swift, Barrett, . . . Weltman. (2008). *Medicine & Science in Sports & Exercise*, *40*(11), 1863.

157 Gutin, B., Barbeau, P., Owens, S., Lemmon, C.R., Bauman, M., Allison, J., . . . Litaker, M.S. (2002). Effects of exercise intensity on cardiovascular fitness, total body composition, and visceral adiposity of obese adolescents. *The American Journal of Clinical Nutrition*, *75*(5), 818–826.

158 Nicklas, Wang, You, Lyles, Demons, Easter, . . . Carr. (2009). *The American Journal of Clinical Nutrition*, *89*(4), 1043–1052.

159 Okura, T., Nakata, Y., & Tanaka, K. (2003). Effects of exercise intensity on physical fitness and risk factors for coronary heart disease. *Obesity Research*, *11*(9), 1131–1139.

160 Pontzer. (2012, August 24). *New York Times.*

161 Tabata, I., Nishimura, K., Kouzaki, M., Hirai, Y., Ogita, F., Miyachi, M., & Yamamoto, K. (1996). Effects of moderate-intensity endurance and high-intensity intermittent training on anaerobic capacity and VO2max. *Medicine & Science in Sports & Exercise, 28*(10), 1327–1330.

162 Boutcher. (2010). *Journal of Obesity, 2011.*

163 Donnelly, J.E., Jacobsen, D.J., Heelan, K.S., Seip, R., & Smith, S. (2000). The effects of 18 months of intermittent vs. continuous exercise on aerobic capacity, body weight and composition, and metabolic fitness in previously sedentary, moderately obese females. *International Journal of Obesity & Related Metabolic Disorders, 24*(5), 566–572.

164 Yoshioka, M., Doucet, E., St-Pierre, S., Almeras, N., Richard, D., Labrie, A., . . . Tremblay, A. (2001). Impact of high-intensity exercise on energy expenditure, lipid oxidation and body fatness. *International Journal of Obesity & Related Metabolic Disorders, 25*(3), 332–339.

165 Bagley, L., Slevin, M., Bradburn, S., Liu, D., Murgatroyd, C., Morrissey, G., . . . McPhee, J.S. (2016). Sex differences in the effects of 12 weeks sprint interval training on body fat mass and the rates of fatty acid oxidation and VO2max during exercise. *BMJ Open Sport & Exercise Medicine, 2*(1), e000056.

166 van Gent, R.N., Siem, D., van Middelkoop, M., van Os, A.G., Bierma-Zeinstra, S.M.A., & Koes, B.W. (2007). Incidence and determinants of lower-extremity running injuries in long distance runners: a systematic review. *British Journal of Sports Medicine, 41*(8), 469–480.

167 Seibert, G. (2013, February). Customer review. Retrieved from: www.amazon.com/Aerobics-Kenneth-H-Cooper/dp/B0006BRNHQ

168 van Gent, Siem, van Middelkoop, van Os, Bierma-Zeinstra, & Koes. (2007). *British Journal of Sports Medicine, 41*(8), 469–480.

169 Nicholl, J.P., & Williams, B. T. (1982). Popular marathons: forecasting casualties. *British Medical Journal* (Clinical Research Ed), *285*(6353), 1464–1465.

170 Davis, I.S., Bowser, B.J., & Mullineaux, D.R. (2015). Reduced vertical impact loading in female runners with medically diagnosed injuries: a prospective investigation. *British Journal of Sports Medicine.* doi: 10.1136/bjsports-2015-094579

171 Reynolds, G. (2016, February 10). Why we get running injuries (and how to prevent them). *New York Times.* Retrieved from: http://well.blogs.nytimes.com/2016/02/10/why-we-get-running-injuries-and-how-to-prevent-them

172 Taunton, J.E., Ryan, M.B., Clement, D.B., McKenzie, D.C., Lloyd-Smith, D.R., & Zumbo, B.D. (2002). A retrospective case-control analysis of 2002 running injuries. *British Journal of Sports Medicine, 36*(2), 95–101.

173 Harper, N. (2016, February 20). Meet the streakers who just can't stop running. *The Telegraph.* Retrieved from: www.telegraph.co.uk/men/active/meet-the-streakers-who-just-cant-stop-running

174 Dahl, M. (2015, November 17). Weird things happen in the minds of ultramarathoners. *NYMag.com, Science of Us.* Retrieved from: http://nymag.com/scienceofus/2015/11/weird-things-happen-in-the-minds-of-ultrarunners.html

175 Fuss, J., Steinle, J., Bindila, L., Auer, M.K., Kirchherr, H., Lutz, B., & Gass, P. (2015). A runner's high depends on cannabinoid receptors in mice. *Proceedings of the National Academy of Sciences, 112*(42), 13105–13108.

176   Kováč, L. (2012). The biology of happiness. *EMBO Reports, 13*(4), 297–302.

177   Nielsen, R.O., Buist, I., Sørensen, H., Lind, M., & Rasmussen, S. (2012). Training errors and running-related injuries: a systematic review. *International Journal of Sports Physical Therapy, 7*(1), 58–75.

178   Videbæk, S., Bueno, A.M., Nielsen, R.O., & Rasmussen, S. (2015). Incidence of running-related injuries per 1,000 h of running in different types of runners: a systematic review and meta-analysis. *Sports Medicine, 45*(7), 1017–1026.

179   Kim, D., Ko, E.J., Cho, H., Park, S.H., Lee, S.H., Cho, N.G., . . . Yang, D.H. (2015). Spinning-induced rhabdomyolysis: eleven case reports and review of the literature. *Electrolytes & Blood Pressure, 13*(2), 58–61.

180   Rhabdomyolysis. (2015, September 22). In *U.S. National Library of Medicine*. Retrieved from: medlineplus.gov/ency/article/000473.htm

181   Ramme, A.J., Vira, S., Alaia, M.J., Van De Leuv, J., & Rothberg, R.C. (Epub 2015, February 10). Exertional rhabdomyolysis after spinning: case series and review of the literature. *The Journal of Sports Medicine and Physical Fitness.*

182   Skoluda, N., Dettenborn, L., Stalder, T., & Kirschbaum, C. (2012). Elevated hair cortisol concentrations in endurance athletes. *Psychoneuroendocrinology, 37*(5), 611–617.

183   Flier, J.S., Harris, M., & Hollenberg, A.N. (2000). Leptin, nutrition, and the thyroid: the why, the wherefore, and the wiring. *Journal of Clinical Investigation, 105*(7), 859–861.

184   Baylor, L.S., & Hackney, A.C. (2003). Resting thyroid and leptin hormone changes in women following intense, prolonged exercise training. *European Journal of Applied Physiology, 88*(4–5), 480–484.

185   American College of Sports Medicine. (2011). The female athlete triad. Retrieved from: www.acsm.org/docs/brochures/the-female-athlete-triad.pdf

186   Ibid.

187   Ellison, P.T. (2003). Energetics and reproductive effort. *American Journal of Human Biology, 15*(3), 342–351.

188   Crouse, L. (2016, January 15). His strength sapped, top marathoner Ryan Hall decides to stop. *New York Times.* Retrieved from: www.nytimes.com/2016/01/17/sports/ryan-hall-fastest-us-distance-runner-is-retiring.html

189   Strout, E. (2016, January 18). Ryan Hall: "our days feel so good and full." *Runners World.* Retrieved from: www.runnersworld.com/elite-runners/ryan-hall-our-days-feel-so-good-and-full

190   Daly, W., Seegers, C.A., Rubin, D.A., Dobridge, J.D., & Hackney, A.C. (2005). Relationship between stress hormones and testosterone with prolonged endurance exercise. *European Journal of Applied Physiology, 93*(4), 375–380.

191   O'Keefe, Schnohr, & Lavie. (2013). *Heart, 99*(8), 588–590.

192   Helliker, K. (2012, November 27). One running shoe in the grave. *Wall Street Journal.* Retrieved from: www.wsj.com/articles/SB10001424127887323330604578145462264024472

193   Harris, K.M., Henry, J.T., Rohman, E., Haas, T.S., & Maron, B.J. (2010). Sudden death during the triathlon. *JAMA, 303*(13), 1255–1257.

194   Farrell, S. (2012, June 25). Aerobic exercise: is more necessarily better? *The Cooper Institute.* Retrieved from: www.cooperinstitute.org/2012/06/aerobic-exercise-is-more-necessarily-better

195 European Society of Cardiology (ESC). (2012, May 3). Regular jogging shows dramatic increase in life expectancy. Retrieved from: www.escardio.org/The-ESC/Press-Office/Press-releases/Regular-jogging-shows-dramatic-increase-in-life-expectancy

196 Statista. (2015). Number of joggers and runners in the U.S.A., 2015. Retrieved from: www.statista.com/statistics/227423/number-of-joggers-and-runners-usa

197 Statista. (2016). Most popular outdoor activities in the U.S. from 2009 to 2013. Retrieved from: www.statista.com/statistics/190202/number-of-participants-in-outdoor-activities-in-the-us-2009

198 Ingraham, P. (2015, October 7). Running on pavement is risky. *Pain Science*. Retrieved from: www.painscience.com/articles/running-on-pavement-is-risky.php

199 Ambros-Rudolph, C.M., Hofmann-Wellenhof, R., Richtig, E., Müller-Fürstner, M., Soyer, H.P., & Kerl, H. (2006). Malignant melanoma in marathon runners. *Archives of Dermatology*, 142(11), 1471–1474.

200 Cacciola, S. (2015, November 2). Unofficially 49,467th, but first among the New York City Marathon's "almost" crew. *New York Times*. Retrieved from: www.nytimes.com/2015/11/03/sports/completing-the-new-york-city-marathon-even-after-the-finish-line-comes-down.html

201 Wansink, B. (2007). *Mindless eating: why we eat more than we think*. Bantam.

202 Rosenbrock, K. (2014, October 29). How many calories does running a marathon burn? *Active Times*. Retrieved from: www.theactivetimes.com/how-many-calories-does-running-marathon-burn.

203 Brown, R.E., Canning, K.L., Fung, M., Jiandani, D., Riddell, M.C., Macpherson, A.K., & Kuk, J.L. (2016). Calorie estimation in adults differing in body weight class and weight loss status. *Medicine & Science in Sports & Exercise*, 48(3), 521–526.

204 Ballantyne, C. (n.d.) Pepperoni pizza 1 – Craig 0 (watch Craig Ballantyne get his butt whooped!). *Early to Rise*. Retrieved from: www.earlytorise.com/cardio-diet-fat-loss/

205 Graybosch, G., Verducci, F., Kern, M., & Lee, C.M. (2011). Accuracy of estimated energy expenditure from the caloric display of an elliptical trainer. *Medicine & Science in Sports & Exercise*, 43(5), 474–475.

206 Smith, J. (n.d.). How (in)accurate are calorie counters at the gym? *Shape*. Retrieved from: www.shape.com/fitness/cardio/how-inaccurate-are-calorie-counters-gym

207 Neff, J., Verona, M., & Roane, J. (2009). Patent U.S. 7497807 B2. Retrieved from: www.google.com/patents/US7497807

208 Dohle, S., Wansink, B., & Zehnder, L. (2015). Exercise and food compensation: exploring diet-related beliefs and behaviors of regular exercisers. *Journal of Physical Activity and Health*, 12(3), 322–327.

209 Wood, P.D., Haskell, W.L., Terry, R.B., Ho, P.H., & Blair, S.N. (1982). Effects of a two-year running program on plasma lipoproteins, body fat and dietary intake in initially sedentary men. *Medicine & Science in Sports & Exercise*, 14(2), 104.

210 Pomerleau, M., Imbeault, P., Parker, T., & Doucet, E. (2004). Effects of exercise intensity on food intake and appetite in women. *The American Journal of Clinical Nutrition*, 80(5), 1230–1236.

211 Elder, S.J., & Roberts, S.B. (2007). The effects of exercise on food intake and body fatness: a summary of published studies. *Nutrition Reviews*, 65(1), 1–19.

212 Wansink, B., & Sobal, J. (2007). Mindless eating: the 200 daily food decisions we overlook. *Environment and Behavior, 39*(1), 106–123.

213 Dohle, Wansink, & Zehnder. (2015). *Journal of Physical Activity and Health, 12*(3), 322–327.

214 Wansink, B. (n.d.). Fueled by treats: exercisers frequently reward themselves with food. Retrieved from: http://foodpsychology.cornell.edu/discoveries/fueled-treats

215 Conroy, D.E., Ram, N., Pincus, A.L., Coffman, D.L., Lorek, A.E., Rebar, A.L., & Roche, M.J. (2015). Daily physical activity and alcohol use across the adult lifespan. *Health Psychology, 34*(6), 653–660.

216 Werle, C.O., Wansink, B., & Payne, C.R. (2011). Just thinking about exercise makes me serve more food: physical activity and calorie compensation. *Appetite, 56*(2), 332–335.

217 Cornell University Food and Brand Lab. (n.d.). Is it fun or exercise? The framing of physical activity biases subsequent snacking. Retrieved from: http://foodpsychology.cornell.edu/research/it-fun-or-exercise-framing-physical-activity-biases-subsequent-snacking

218 Kennedy, M.A., Sacheck, J., Folta, S.C., Houser, R., Kuder, J., & Nelson, M.E. (2010). The impact of marathon training on body weight in recreational runners: 2436: board 44, June 4, 8:00 a.m.–9:30 a.m. *Medicine & Science in Sports & Exercise, 42*(5), 625.

219 Westerterp, K.R., Meijer, G.A., Janssen, E.M., Saris, W.H., & Ten Hoor, F. (1992). Long-term effect of physical activity on energy balance and body composition. *British Journal of Nutrition, 68*(01), 21–30.

220 Janssen, Graef, & Saris. (1989). *International Journal of Sports Medicine, 10*(suppl 1), S17–21.

221 Pontzer, Durazo-Arvizu, Dugas, Plange-Rhule, Bovet, Forrester, . . . & Luke. (2016). *Current Biology, 26*(3), 410–417.

222 Drenowatz, C., Grieve, G.L., & DeMello, M.M. (2015). Change in energy expenditure and physical activity in response to aerobic and resistance exercise programs. *SpringerPlus, 4*(1), 1–9.

223 Biswas, A., Oh, P.I., Faulkner, G.E., Bajaj, R.R., Silver, M.A., Mitchell, M.S., & Alter, D.A. (2015). Sedentary time and its association with risk for disease incidence, mortality, and hospitalization in adults: a systematic review and meta-analysis. *Annals of Internal Medicine, 162*(2), 123–132.

224 Williams, P.T. (2005). Nonlinear relationships between weekly walking distance and adiposity in 27,596 women. *Medicine & Science in Sports & Exercise, 37*(11), 1893–1901.

225 Williams, P.T. (2007). Self-selection contributes significantly to the lower adiposity of faster, longer-distanced, male and female walkers. *International Journal of Obesity, 31*(4), 652–662.

226 Tremblay, Després, Leblanc, Craig, Ferris, Stephens, & Bouchard. (1990). *The American Journal of Clinical Nutrition, 51*(2), 153–157.

227 Clemens, L.H., Slawson, D.L., & Klesges, R.C. (1999). The effect of eating out on quality of diet in premenopausal women. *Journal of the American Dietetic Association, 99*(4), 442–444.

228 Guthrie, J.F., Lin, B.H., & Frazao, E. (2002). Role of food prepared away from home in the American diet, 1977–78 versus 1994–96: changes and consequences. *Journal of Nutrition Education and Behavior, 34*(3), 140–150.

229 Wansink, B. (n.d.) Fueled by treats: exercisers frequently reward themselves with food. Retrieved from: http://foodpsychology.cornell.edu/discoveries/fueled-treats

230 Janssen, I., Heymsfield, S.B., Wang, Z.M., & Ross, R. (2000). Skeletal muscle mass and distribution in 468 men and women aged 18–88 yr. *Journal of Applied Physiology, 89*(1), 81–88.

231 Ballor, D.L., & Keesey, R.E. (1991). A meta-analysis of the factors affecting exercise-induced changes in body mass, fat mass and fat-free mass in males and females. *International Journal of Obesity, 15*(11), 717–726.

232 Garrow, & Summerbell. (1995). *European Journal of Clinical Nutrition, 49*(1), 1–10.

233 Bryner, Ullrich, Sauers, Donley, Hornsby, Kolar, & Yeater. (1999). *Journal of the American College of Nutrition, 18*(2), 115–121.

234 National Center for Health Statistics. (2015, May). Health, United States, 2014: with special feature on adults aged 55–64. Report No. 2015-1232. Hyattsville, MD.

235 Smith, G.S., Wellman, H.M., Sorock, G.S., Warner, M., Courtney, T.K., Pransky, G.S., & Fingerhut, L.A. (2005). Injuries at work in the U.S. adult population: contributions to the total injury burden. *American Journal of Public Health, 95*(7), 1213–1219.

236 van Gent, Siem, van Middelkoop, van Os, Bierma-Zeinstra, & Koes. (2007). *British Journal of Sports Medicine, 41*(8), 469–480.

237 Lustig, R.H. (2012). *Fat chance: beating the odds against sugar, processed food, obesity, and disease.* Hudson Street Press.

238 Hall, K.D., Sacks, G., Chandramohan, D., Chow, C.C., Wang, Y.C., Gortmaker, S.L., & Swinburn, B.A. (2011). Quantification of the effect of energy imbalance on bodyweight. *The Lancet, 378*(9793), 826–837.

239 Lustig. (2012). Hudson Street Press.

240 Ballor, & Keesey. (1991). *International Journal of Obesity, 15*(11), 717–726.

241 Garrow, & Summerbell. (1995). *European Journal of Clinical Nutrition, 49*(1), 1–10.

242 Drenowatz, C., Hand, G.A., Sagner, M., Shook, R.P., Burgess, S., & Blair, S.N. (2015). The prospective association between different types of exercise and body composition. *Medicine & Science in Sports & Exercise, 47*(12), 2535–2541.

243 Westcott, W.L. (2012). Resistance training is medicine: effects of strength training on health. *Current Sports Medicine Reports, 11*(4), 209–216.

244 Lustig. (2012). Penguin.

245 Ibañez, J., Izquierdo, M., Argüelles, I., Forga, L., Larrión, J.L., García-Unciti, M., . . . Gorostiaga, E.M. (2005). Twice-weekly progressive resistance training decreases abdominal fat and improves insulin sensitivity in older men with type 2 diabetes. *Diabetes Care, 28*(3), 662–667.

246 Hunter, G.R., Byrne, N.M., Sirikul, B., Fernández, J.R., Zuckerman, P.A., Darnell, B.E., & Gower, B.A. (2008). Resistance training conserves fat-free mass and resting energy expenditure following weight loss. *Obesity, 16*(5), 1045–1051.

247 Iglay, H.B., Thyfault, J.P., Apolzan, J.W. & Campbell W.W. (2007). Resistance training and dietary protein: effects on glucose tolerance and contents of skeletal muscle insulin signaling proteins in older persons. *American Journal of Clinical Nutrition 85*(4), 1005–1013.

248 Kennedy, J.F. (1962, July 16). Article by the president: the vigor we need. *Sports Illustrated.* Retrieved from: www.presidency.ucsb.edu/ws/?pid=8771

249 Bryner, Ullrich, Sauers, Donley, Hornsby, Kolar, & Yeater. (1999). *Journal of the American College of Nutrition, 18*(2), 115–121.

250 Kerksick, C.M., Wilborn, C.D., Campbell, B.I., Roberts, M.D., Rasmussen, C.J., Greenwood, M., & Kreider, R.B. (2009). Early-phase adaptations to a split-body, linear periodization resistance training program in college-aged and middle-aged men. *The Journal of Strength & Conditioning Research, 23*(3), 962–971.

251 Ibañez, Izquierdo, Argüelles, Forga, Larrión, García-Unciti, . . . Gorostiaga. (2005). *Diabetes Care, 28*(3), 662–667.

252 Ibid.

253 Cooper, K.H. (1968). *Aerobics*. New York: M. Evans and Co.

254 Voelker, R. (2008, Fall). Measuring fitness today. *CooperHealth*. Retrieved from: www.cooperaerobics.com/Downloads/About/CooperHealth_F08_FINAL.aspx

255 Cleveland Clinic Heart and Vascular Team. (2014, January 8). Four surprising heart attack triggers. Retrieved from: https://health.clevelandclinic.org/2014/01/surprising-heart-attack-triggers

256 Griffin, R.M. (2013, October 14). Myths about exercise and older adults. *WebMD Feature*. Retrieved from: www.webmd.com/healthy-aging/nutrition-world-2/exercise-older-adults

257 Willson, J.D., Dougherty, C.P., Ireland, M.L., & Davis, I.M. (2005). Core stability and its relationship to lower extremity function and injury. *Journal of the American Academy of Orthopaedic Surgeons*, 13(5), 316–325.

258 Roizen, M. (2015, October 26). Four simple ways to get healthier without going to extremes. *Robb Report*. Retrieved from: http://robbreport.com/health-and-wellness/living-well/four-simple-ways-get-healthier-without-going-extremes/page/0/1

259 Janssen, Heymsfield, Wang, & Ross. (2000). *Journal of Applied Physiology*, 89(1), 81–88.

260 Ballor, & Keesey. (1991). *International Journal of Obesity*, 15(11), 717–726.

261 National Center for Health Statistics. (2105). Hyattsville, MD.

262 Bush, C. (2012, April 20). Your guide to exercising through the ages. *U.S. News*. Retrieved from: http://health.usnews.com/health-news/articles/2012/04/20/your-guide-to-exercising-through-the-ages

263 Lemes, Í.R., Ferreira, P.H., Linares, S.N., Machado, A.F., Pastre, C.M., & Netto, J. (2016). Resistance training reduces systolic blood pressure in metabolic syndrome: a systematic review and meta-analysis of randomised controlled trials. *British Journal of Sports Medicine*, pii: bjsports-2015-094715. doi: 10.1136/bjsports-2015-094715

264 Paffenbarger Jr, & Hale. (1975). *New England Journal of Medicine*, 292(11), 545–550.

265 Hallsworth, K., Fattakhova, G., Hollingsworth, K.G., Thoma, C., Moore, S., Taylor, R., . . . Trenell, M.I. (2011). Resistance exercise reduces liver fat and its mediators in non-alcoholic fatty liver disease independent of weight loss. *Gut*, 60(9), 1278–1283.

266 National Heart, Lung, and Blood Institute. (n.d.). What is metabolic syndrome? Retrieved from: www.nhlbi.nih.gov/health/health-topics/topics/ms

267 Albright, A., Franz, M., Hornsby, G., Kriska, A., Marrero, D., Ullrich, I., & Verity, L.S. (2000). American college of sports medicine position stand. Exercise and type 2 diabetes. *Medicine & Science in Sports & Exercise*, 32(7), 1345–1360.

268 Ibañez, Izquierdo, Argüelles, Forga, Larrión, García-Unciti, . . . Gorostiaga. (2005). *Diabetes Care*, 28(3), 662–667.

269 Lee, I.M. (2003). Physical activity and cancer prevention—data from epidemiologic studies. *Medicine & Science in Sports & Exercise*, 35(11), 1823–1827.

270 Lynch, B.M., Neilson, H.K., & Friedenreich, C.M. (2010). Physical activity and breast cancer prevention. In *Physical Activity and Cancer* (pp. 13-42). Springer Berlin Heidelberg.

271 American Council on Exercise. (2013, April). ACE-sponsored research study: kettlebells kick butt. Retrieved from: www.acefitness.org/certifiednewsarticle/3172/ace-sponsored-research-study-kettlebells-kick-butt

272 American Council on Exercise. (2010, February 8). Press release: ACE study reveals kettlebells provide powerful workout in short amount of time. Retrieved from: www.acefitness.org/about-ace/press-room/528/ace-study-reveals-kettlebells-provide-powerful

273 Farrar, R.E., Mayhew, J.L., & Koch, A.J. (2010). Oxygen cost of kettlebell swings. *The Journal of Strength & Conditioning Research, 24*(4), 1034–1036.

274 Harrison, J.S., Schoenfeld, B., & Schoenfeld, M.L. (2011). Applications of kettlebells in exercise program design. *Strength & Conditioning Journal, 33*(6), 86–89.

275 Williams, P.T., & Wood, P.D. (2006). The effects of changing exercise levels on weight and age-related weight gain. *International Journal of Obesity, 30*(3), 543–551.

276 Gilbert, K. (2015, October 29). And the biggest fitness trends in 2016 will be . . . *Shape.* Retrieved from: www.shape.com/fitness/workouts/and-biggest-fitness-trends-2016-will-be

277 McRae, G., Payne, A., Zelt, J.G., Scribbans, T.D., Jung, M.E., Little, J.P., & Gurd, B.J. (2012). Extremely low-volume, whole-body aerobic–resistance training improves aerobic fitness and muscular endurance in females. *Applied Physiology, Nutrition, and Metabolism, 37*(6), 1124–1131.

278 Bagley, L., Slevin, M., Bradburn, S., Liu, D., Murgatroyd, C., Morrissey, G., . . . McPhee, J.S. (2016). Sex differences in the effects of 12 weeks of sprint interval training on body fat mass and the rates of fatty acid oxidation and VO2max during exercise. *BMJ Open Sport & Exercise Medicine, 2*(1), e000056. doi: 10.1136/bjmsm-2015-000056

279 Gillen, J.B., Martin, B.J., MacInnis, M.J., Skelly, L.E., Tarnopolsky, M.A., & Gibala, M.J. (2016). Twelve weeks of sprint interval training improves indices of cardiometabolic health similar to traditional endurance training despite a five-fold lower exercise volume and time commitment. *PloS One, 11*(4), e0154075. doi: 10.1371/journal.pone.0154075

280 Trapp, Chisholm, Freund, & Boutcher. (2008). *International Journal of Obesity, 32*(4), 684–691.

281 Little, J.P., Gillen, J.B., Percival, M.E., Safdar, A., Tarnopolsky, M.A., Punthakee, Z., . . . Gibala, M.J. (2011). Low-volume high-intensity interval training reduces hyperglycemia and increases muscle mitochondrial capacity in patients with type 2 diabetes. *Journal of Applied Physiology, 111*(6), 1554–1560.

282 Borg, G.A. (1982). Psychophysical bases of perceived exertion. *Medicine & Science in Sports & Exercise, 14*(5), 377–381.

283 Mata, J., Todd, P.M., & Lippke, S. (2010). When weight management lasts. Lower perceived rule complexity increases adherence. *Appetite, 54*(1), 37–43.

284 Guthrie, Lin, & Frazao. (2002). *Journal of Nutrition Education and Behavior, 34*(3), 140–150.

285 United States Department of Agriculture, Office of Communications. (March 2003). *Agriculture fact book 2001-2002.*

286 Clemens, Slawson, & Klesges. (1999). *Journal of the American Dietetic Association, 99*(4), 442–444.

287 Guthrie, Lin, & Frazao. (2002). *Journal of Nutrition Education and Behavior, 34*(3), 140–150.

288 French, S.A., Story, M., & Jeffery, R.W. (2001). Environmental influences on eating and physical activity. *Annual Review of Public Health, 22*(1), 309–335.

289 Johnson, R.K., Appel, L.J., Brands, M., Howard, B.V., Lefevre, M., Lustig, R.H., . . . Wylie-Rosett, J.

(2009). Dietary sugars intake and cardiovascular health: a scientific statement from the American Heart Association. *Circulation,* *120*(11), 1011–1020.

290 Kaiser Permanente. (2008, July 8). Keeping a food diary doubles diet weight loss, study suggests. *ScienceDaily*. Retrieved from: www.sciencedaily.com/releases/2008/07/080708080738.htm

291 Shay, C.M., Van Horn, L., Stamler, J., Dyer, A.R., Brown, I.J., Chan, Q., . . . Elliott, P. (2012). Food and nutrient intakes and their associations with lower BMI in middle-aged U.S. adults: the international study of macro-/micronutrients and blood pressure (INTERMAP). *The American Journal of Clinical Nutrition, 96*(3), 483–491.

292 Ello-Martin, J.A., Roe, L.S., Ledikwe, J.H., Beach, A.M., & Rolls, B.J. (2007). Dietary energy density in the treatment of obesity: a yearlong trial comparing 2 weight-loss diets. *The American Journal of Clinical Nutrition, 85*(6), 1465–1477.

293 Mattes, R.D., Kris-Etherton, P.M., & Foster, G.D. (2008). Impact of peanuts and tree nuts on body weight and healthy weight loss in adults. *The Journal of Nutrition, 138*(9), 1741S–1745S.

294 Garciá-Lorda, P., Rangil, I.M., & Salas-Salvadó, J. (2003). Nut consumption, body weight, and insulin resistance. *European Journal of Clinical Nutrition, 57*(suppl 1), S8–S11.

295 Wien, M.A., Sabaté, J.M., Iklé, D.N., Cole, S.E., & Kandeel, F.R. (2003). Almonds vs. complex carbohydrates in a weight reduction program. *International Journal of Obesity and Related Metabolic Disorders, 27*(11), 1365–1372.

296 Shai, I., Schwarzfuchs, D., Henkin, Y., Shahar, D.R., Witkow, S., Greenberg, I., . . . Stampfer, M.J. (2008). Weight loss with a low-carbohydrate, Mediterranean, or low-fat diet. *New England Journal of Medicine, 359*(3), 229–241.

297 Stookey, J.D., Constant, F., Popkin, B.M., & Gardner, C.D. (2008). Drinking water is associated with weight loss in overweight dieting women independent of diet and activity. *Obesity, 16*(11), 2481–2488.

298 Shay, Van Horn, Stamler, Dyer, Brown, Chan, . . . Elliott. (2012). *The American Journal of Clinical Nutrition, 96*(3), 483–491.

299 Thompson, P.L. (2013). J-curve revisited: cardiovascular benefits of moderate alcohol use cannot be dismissed. *The Medical Journal of Australia, 198*(8), 419–422.

300 Johnson, Appel, Brands, Howard, Lefevre, Lustig, . . . Wylie-Rosett. (2009). *Circulation, 120*(11), 1011–1020.

301 Ibid.

302 Liu, S., Willett, W.C., Stampfer, M.J., Hu, F.B., Franz, M., Sampson, L., . . . Manson, J.E. (2000). A prospective study of dietary glycemic load, carbohydrate intake, and risk of coronary heart disease in US women. *The American Journal of Clinical Nutrition, 71*(6), 1455–1461.

303 Johnson, Appel, Brands, Howard, Lefevre, Lustig, . . . Wylie-Rosett. (2009). *Circulation, 120*(11), 1011–1020.

304 Shai, Schwarzfuchs, Henkin, Shahar, Witkow, Greenberg, . . . Tangi-Rozental. (2008). *New England Journal of Medicine, 359*(3), 229–241.

305 Liu, Willett, Stampfer, Hu, Franz, Sampson, . . . Manson. (2000). *The American Journal of Clinical Nutrition, 71*(6), 1455–1461.

ACKNOWLEDGMENTS

The authors would like to acknowledge the extraordinary support of Jill Alexander at Quarto Publishing Group who championed this book from the beginning and suggested valuable improvements along the way. It is also vastly better because of the thoughtful, detailed review and comments of Julia Gaviria, and the careful copyediting of Mary Cassells.

Craig would also like to thank Lou Schuler and Adam Campbell for giving him his big break when they took a chance and published a young, outspoken personal trainer's advice that would go on to change the fitness world.

ABOUT THE AUTHORS

CRAIG BALLANTYNE

Craig Ballantyne is a Productivity and Success Transformation Coach from Toronto, Ontario, Canada, and the author of *The Perfect Day Formula: How to Own the Day and Control Your Life.*

He has been a contributor to *Men's Health* magazine since 2000, and his articles have also appeared in *Women's Health, Oxygen, GQ, Maxim, National Geographic, Men's Fitness,* and *Muscle & Fitness Hers,* among many others. His articles have also been featured on inc.com, lifehacker.com, and telegraph.co.uk.

In 2001, Craig created the popular home workout program, Turbulence Training (turbulancetraining.com), and in 2013 he created the Home Workout Revolution bodyweight exercise program (homeworkoutrevolution.com). Over 100,000 men and women have used his 6 Minutes to Skinny weight loss system since 2014.

Craig is also the founder of the Certified Turbulence Training Program, certifying trainers from all corners of the globe. He holds an annual Turbulence Training Summit every year for fitness experts to become better trainers.

Craig's online success has led him to create books and a coaching program to show other gurus how to take their ideas and help thousands of people. He holds seminars around the world, and he teaches at the annual Sovereign Academy camp every summer in Lithuania.

Craig has had to overcome many obstacles on his journey to success, and his toughest battle was fighting crippling anxiety attacks. He finally discovered how to beat them with his 5 Pillars of Transformation, and, today, Craig shows men and women how to use the 5 Pillars to lose 10 to 75 pounds (4.5 to 34 kg), get a raise and make more money, find the love of their life, and overcome any obstacle in the way of success. On his website, earlytorise.com, you'll find his daily essays on success, productivity, time management, fitness, weight loss, and self-improvement.

CHELSEA RATCLIFF

Chelsea Ratcliff is a graduate student in health communication. She is specializing in how health research is employed by health professionals and the media to guide health-based behaviors and recommendations. She has been a freelance health and fitness writer since 2009, writing for several outlets including *U.S. News & World Report*. She lives in Salt Lake City, Utah. Follow her peer-reviewed research and journalism articles at www.chelsearatcliff.com and on Twitter at @chelseawriting.

INDEX

metabolic resistance training (MRT)
  afterburn and, 147
  Cross-Body Mountain Climber, 149
  Dumbbell Row, 150
  Dumbbell Split Squat, 154
  Goblet Squat, 148
  introduction to, 147
  Kettlebell Swing, 152
  One-Arm Standing Dumbbell Press, 155
  Plank, 151
  Push-up, 153
metabolism
  basal metabolic rate, 36, 42, 68
  behavioral compensation effect, 107
  compensation mechanisms, 103–105, 107, 108
  definition of, 68
  energy expenditure ceiling, 107
  metabolic syndrome, 122, 123
  middle age and, 116
  muscle and, 38, 42, 43, 68, 116
  physiological compensation effect, 107
  strength training and, 117
  testosterone and, 40
  thermogenesis, 68
middle age
  Body Mass Index (BMI) and, 113
  deaths, 48, 51
  exertion deaths, 120
  interval training and, 37, 38
  kettlebell workouts and, 124
  metabolism and, 116, 123
  muscle and, 115–116, 118
  risk factors and, 123
  strength training and, 38, 113
  weight loss and, 114–117
Morris, Jerry, 48
Mountain Climber workout, 141
multitasking, 67, 69
muscle
  age and, 118
  amino acids and, 41–42
  calories and, 42

core muscles, 124
glycogen and, 77
injuries and, 85
intensity and, 74
intervals and, 77
metabolism and, 35, 37, 38, 42, 43, 68
middle age and, 115–116, 118
rhabdomyolysis, 89
strength training and, 115

N

National Institutes of Health (NIH), 9
New England Journal of Medicine, 48
New York Times newspaper, 9, 10, 86
Nurses' Health Study, 60, 164
nutrition. See also calories.
  alcoholic drinks, 46, 164
  American diet, 158–159, 163
  calories and, 100
  cheese, 158
  coffee, 163
  environment and, 165
  fast food, 158–159
  female athlete triad and, 91
  food journaling, 160
  fruits, 162
  habits for, 165
  meats, 163
  nuts, 162–163
  processed carbohydrates, 164–165
  sample menu, 161
  sugar, 164
  tea, 163
  vegetables, 162
  water, 163
  women and, 161, 164
nuts, 162–163

O

Obesity journal, 22
O'Keefe, James, 59, 92

One-Arm Standing Dumbbell Press workout, 155

P

Pheidippides, 92
physiological compensation effect, 107
Pilon, Brad, 100
Plank workout, 151
plateaus, 130
Pontzer, Herman, 71–72, 74, 76, 78
Porcari, John, 124
Prisoner Squat workout, 133
processed carbohydrates, 164–165
Punisher Squat workout, 145
Purdue University, 116
Push-up workout, 153

R

Ratcliff, Chelsea, 8
Rating of Perceived Exertion (RPE) Scale, 144
resistance training. *See* strength training.
Reynolds, Gretchen, 86
rhabdomyolysis, 89
risk factors
  cancer, 33, 123
  Copenhagen City Heart Study, 53–54
  diabetes, 33, 123
  heart disease, 53–54
  metabolic syndrome, 123
  middle age and, 123
Rocking Plank workout, 139
Romanov, Nicholas, 88
Runner's World magazine, 91
running. *See also* marathons.
  air quality and, 93
  Copenhagen City Heart Study, 58–59
  deaths and, 19, 45, 51, 58, 59, 92
  "dosage" of, 58–59
  euphoria and, 87–88
  injuries from, 69, 84, 85, 88–89

International Marathon
 (Baghdad), 53
long-term results of, 83–84
popularity of, 19
self-selection bias, 104
skin cancer and, 93
skinny runners, 104
"streaking," 86
triathlons, 92–93
The Running Revolution
 (Nicholas Romanov), 88
*Running and Being: The Total
 Experience* (George Sheehan), 50

S

Schnohr, Peter, 58, 59, 93
self-selection bias, 104
Sheehan, George, 18, 19, 50
Shmerling, Robert H., 51
Simmons, Richard, 19
skin cancer, 93
smoking, 20, 33, 46, 53
"The Soft American" (John F.
 Kennedy), 15, 19, 26, 117
Solomon, Henry, 57, 58, 87
Sorlie, Paul, 54
Spiderman Push-up, 134
spinning, injuries from, 89
Sports Illustrated magazine, 15, 26
Sports Medicine journal, 88
stages of grief, 47
steady-state exercise (SSE), 37, 43
"streak" running, 86
strength training
    aerobic exercise and, 24,
     25–26, 37–38
    combined aerobics-and-
     strength-training program, 38
    daily activity and, 105, 106
    dangers of, 26–27
    definition of, 18
    diabetes and, 55, 116, 118–119,
     122, 123
    guidelines for, 121
    health benefits of, 122
    human nature and, 67
    injury resistance and, 120

intensity and, 118
kettlebell workouts, 122, 124
metabolism and, 117
middle age and, 113
muscle and, 115
safety of, 119–120
studies of, 34–36
weight loss and, 34-36, 38, 116
women and, 120–122
stress
    cortisol and, 90
    life span and, 87
    stress tests, 57, 119–120
subcutaneous fat, 33, 35, 70
sugar, 164
Switzer, Kathrine, 26

T

Tabata, Izumi, 36, 76
tea, 163
testosterone, 40, 91–92
thermogenesis, 68
Total Body Extension workout,
 136, 138
Trapp, Ethlyn, 36, 143
treadmill, binge-to-workout
 bargain and, 101–102
Tremblay, Angelo, 34, 41, 70
triathlons, 92–93
True, Micah, 47, 51, 57, 58
Turbulence Training program, 8, 78

U

United States Department of
 Agriculture (USDA), 33
United States National Library of
 Medicine, 89
University of Leeds, 40
University of Oklahoma, 118
University of Wisconsin–La
 Crosse, 122, 124

V

visceral fat, 33, 39, 55, 70, 122, 159

W

Wake Forest University School of
 Medicine, 73
Wansink, Brian, 99, 101, 108
warm-ups, 130–131
water, 163
weightlifting. *See* strength
 training.
weight loss. *See also* fat.
    aerobic exercise and, 21–23, 29
    body composition and, 39
    Body Mass Index (BMI), 39
    deaths and, 20
    exercise intensity and, 73–74
    fat-burning zone, 75
    growth hormone and, 77
    intensity and, 76
    interval training and, 22, 25,
     34–36, 36–37, 41, 69–70, 77, 143
    middle age and, 114–117
    motivation and, 31
    obesity rates, 23
    steady-state exercise (SSE)
     and, 37, 43
    strength training and, 34–36,
     38, 116
Westcott, Wayne, 116
West Virginia University, 37–38
women
    calorie requirements, 161
    cancer and, 123
    cardiovascular disease (CVD)
     and, 60
    Copenhagen City Heart
     Study, 54
    deaths, 51, 54, 60
    estrogen, 60
    female athlete triad, 91
    interval training and, 37, 38
    leptin and, 90
    marathons and, 26
    nutrition and, 161, 164
    running injuries, 85, 86
    sample menu for, 161
    spinning injuries, 89
    strength training and, 113, 116,
     120–122, 142
    weight loss and, 41, 69, 102–103